Nursing care

In

Vascular Surgery

The Complete Guide

ALEXANDRE CAREWELL

Table of contents

Chapter 1: Introduction to vascular surgery — 15

- History and development of vascular surgery — 15
- The importance of vascular surgery in modern medicine — 16

Chapter 2: Nurses' roles and responsibilities — 19

- Essential clinical functions — 19
- The nurse: the link between the surgeon, the patient and the team — 21
- Stress and emergency management — 23

Chapter 3: Knowledge of vascular anatomy — 25

- Circulatory system: an overview — 25
- Main vessels and their characteristics — 27
- Common vascular anomalies — 29

Chapter 4: Common techniques and procedures — 31

- Basics of vascular surgery — 31

- Assistance during angiography, endarterectomy and other procedures 33
- Post-operative management 34

Chapter 5: Tools and equipment 37

- Introduction to essential tools 37
- Maintenance, sterilisation and precautions 38
- Modern technology and innovation 39

Chapter 6: Interaction with the patient 42

- Preoperative patient assessment 42
- Educating the patient: explanations and reassurance 43
- Post-operative follow-up and rehabilitation 45

Chapter 7: Complication management 48

- Rapid identification of warning signs 48
- Emergency and response protocols 49
- Emotional support for patients and their families 51

Chapter 8: Interprofessional communication 54

- Working with surgeons, anaesthetists and technicians 54
- Sharing information with paramedics 56

- Navigating difficult communication situations   57

Chapter 9: Technological updates and innovations   60

- Latest advances in vascular imaging   60
- Simulations and virtual training for nurses   61
- Telesurgery and telemedicine in vascular surgery   63

Chapter 10: Risk management and patient safety   66

- Identifying and anticipating potential hazards   66
- Safety protocols and checklists   67
- The role of the nurse in improving the quality of care   69

Chapter 11: Pharmacology in vascular surgery   72

- Commonly used drugs and their mechanism of action   72
- Drug interactions and side effects   74
- Post-operative pain management   75

Chapter 12: Ethical challenges specific to vascular surgery   78

- Allocating resources and prioritising patients   78

- Refusal of treatment and patient autonomy — 80
- End of life and vascular surgery — 81

Chapter 13: Prevention and patient education — 84

- Prevention of vascular diseases — 84
- Promoting healthy lifestyles — 86
- Importance of regular monitoring — 87

Chapter 14: Integrating telemedicine — 89

- Usefulness and effectiveness of telemedicine in vascular surgery — 89
- Training and skills required for nurses — 90
- Challenges and benefits of this approach — 92

Chapter 15: Special cases and specific populations — 94

- Paediatric vascular surgery: specific features and challenges — 94
- Care for the elderly — 96
- Adapting care for at-risk populations — 97

Chapter 16: Emergency vascular surgery — 99

- Recognising a vascular emergency — 99
- Protocols and rapid intervention — 100
- Managing post-emergency recovery — 102

Chapter 17: Palliative care in vascular surgery   104

- When surgery is no longer an option   104
- Psychological support and symptom relief   105
- Working with palliative care teams   107

Chapter 18: Healthcare-associated infections   109

- Infection prevention   109
- Management and treatment of post-operative infections   110
- The challenges of antibiotic resistance   112

Chapter 19: Rapid recovery after surgery (RRAC)   114

- Principles of RRAC in vascular surgery   114
- The key role of the nurse in the RRAC pathway   116
- Benefits and challenges of this approach   117

Chapter 20: The future of vascular surgery: innovations and challenges   119

- New techniques and materials   119
- Vascular surgery in the digital age   120
- Ethical issues surrounding medical innovations   122

Chapter 21: Transition between hospital and home 124

- Discharge planning and patient education 124
- Post-operative monitoring at home 125
- Working with home care and rehabilitation services 127

Chapter 22: Vascular trauma and management 129

- Initial trauma assessment 129
- Emergency response and stabilisation 130
- Post-traumatic recovery and rehabilitation 132

Chapter 23: Digital tools and applications for nurses 134

- Patient monitoring and assessment software 134
- Use of connectedobjects in post-operative monitoring 135
- Digital security and data confidentiality 137

Chapter 24: Specialisations and sub-disciplines in vascular surgery 140

- Angiology and venous pathologies 140
- Endovascular and minimally invasive techniques 141

- The role of the nurse in cardiovascular surgery ... 143

Chapter 25: Patient safety and management of medical errors ... 146

- Preventing errors in vascular surgery ... 146
- Managing and communicating after an error ... 147
- Feedback for continuous improvement ... 149

Chapter 26: Resource management and operational efficiency ... 151

- Optimising patient flows and the use of resources ... 151
- Time and workload management techniques ... 152
- Technology as an efficiency tool ... 154

Chapter 27: The future of vascular surgery: scenarios and projections ... 156

- Technological advances on the horizon ... 156
- Demographic and epidemiological challenges ... 157
- Looking ahead: preparing the nurse of tomorrow ... 159

Chapter 28: Professional development ... 161

- Continuing education and specialisation ... 161
- Interdisciplinary collaboration ... 162

- Research and academic contributions 164

Conclusion: The future of vascular surgery and the role of the nurse 166

- Technological advances and innovations 166
- The changing role of nurses in a changing medical world 167
- Advice for aspiring vascular surgery nurses 169

« Vascular surgery: the art of repairing the body's motorways while avoiding blood clogs ! »

Chapter 1:
INTRODUCTION
VASCULAR SURGERY

History and development of vascular surgery

Vascular surgery, the fascinating medical speciality that focuses on the body's blood vessels, has a rich history that reflects the constant evolution of medicine. To delve into its past is to travel through the ages, from the first primitive incisions to the advanced surgical techniques we know today.

The history of vascular surgery dates back to ancient times. The ancient Egyptians, for example, had already identified and documented vascular diseases in their medical papyri. However, it is Hippocrates, the father of modern medicine, who is often credited with the first descriptions of thrombosis and embolism in the fifth century BC.

As the centuries progressed, iconic figures emerged, leaving an indelible mark on the world of vascular surgery. One notable example is Ambroise Paré, the sixteenth-century French surgeon who, departing from traditional methods, introduced innovative surgical techniques to treat traumatic vascular lesions.

However, it was in the 19th century, with the advent of anaesthesia and improvements in surgical technique, that vascular surgery experienced a significant boom. Surgeons began to explore new techniques for accessing deep vessels and treating various vascular pathologies. The invention of the microscope, for example, revolutionised vascular microsurgery, allowing precise suturing of small vessels.

The twentieth century was marked by rapid technological advances. The introduction of angiography allowed precise visualisation of vessels, paving the way for more targeted interventions. In addition, endovascular surgery, a less invasive method that uses image-guided catheters to treat vascular disorders, transformed the specialty.

Today, at the dawn of the 21st century, vascular surgery continues to reinvent itself. The use of robotics, 3D printing and artificial intelligence promises to push back even further the boundaries of what surgeons can achieve. As we look to the future, it is essential to remember our rich past, for it is by understanding where we have come from that we can best envisage where we are going.

This journey through time shows that vascular surgery has always been at the forefront of medical innovation. Each era has brought its own challenges and solutions, shaping a speciality that continues to evolve and improve the lives of patients around the world.

The importance of vascular surgery in modern medicine

At the heart of the human body lies a complex network of blood vessels that ensure the circulation of blood and, consequently, the distribution of oxygen and nutrients to every organ and tissue. This vascular system, essential to life, is also subject to a variety of pathologies that can seriously compromise an individual's health. Herein lies the fundamental importance of vascular surgery in modern medicine.

Vascular surgery, as a specialised discipline, deals with disorders of the blood vessels, with the exception of those of the heart and brain. The pathologies treated by this speciality are varied and may be congenital, degenerative, inflammatory or even traumatic. The consequences of these conditions can be as benign as a simple varicose vein or as fatal as a ruptured aortic aneurysm.

In modern medicine, the management of these diseases has major implications for public health. For example, atherosclerosis, a degenerative disease of the arteries, is a major cause of morbidity and mortality worldwide, leading to serious conditions such as strokes, heart attacks and limb amputations. Vascular interventions not only save lives but also improve quality of life by reducing pain, improving mobility and avoiding serious complications.

The importance of vascular surgery also extends beyond the treatment of disease. In the world of organ transplantation, for example, mastery of vascular techniques is essential for organ removal and transplantation. Without successful vascular intervention, transplantation of a kidney, liver or other vital organ would be impossible.

Furthermore, with the constant evolution of medical technology, vascular surgery finds itself at the convergence of innovation. Minimally invasive endovascular techniques, for example, have transformed the management of many vascular pathologies, enabling safer interventions, shorter recovery times and reduced scarring for patients.

Vascular surgery is an essential pillar of modern medicine. It meets critical medical needs, influences related medical fields and constantly pushes the boundaries of what is possible in medicine. Recognising its importance means understanding the extent to which the health and well-being of many people depend on the expertise and skills of vascular surgeons.

Chapter 2:
ROLES AND RESPONSIBILITIES THE NURSE

Essential clinical functions

Vascular surgery, with its vital role in the treatment of blood vessel diseases, requires a range of specific skills to ensure optimal patient care. Let's take a look at the essential clinical functions inherent in this speciality.

- Assessment and Diagnosis :
    - Accurate interpretation of vascular symptoms, ranging from pain in the limbs to non-healing wounds.
    - Use of diagnostic imaging, such as Doppler ultrasound, angiography or MRI, to visualise and assess blood vessels.
    - Functional tests, such as pressure measurements to detect constrictions or obstructions.
- Surgical procedures :
    - Traditional open procedures, such as bypasses to bypass diseased arterial segments.
    - Less invasive endovascular techniques, such as angioplasty and stenting.
    - Aneurysm surgery, in particular endovascular aortic aneurysm repair (EVAR).
    - Procedures for venous disease, including venous stripping and ablations.
- Emergency management :
    - Management of vascular emergencies such as ruptured aneurysms or arterial embolisms.
    - Rapid intervention for acute ischaemia, minimising the risk of limb loss.

- Post-operative care :
  - Close monitoring of patients to detect early complications after surgery.
  - Managing pain, wounds and any infections.
  - Assessment of the perfusion of the operated limbs to ensure optimum circulation.
- Advice and prevention:
  - Patient education on vascular risk factors, including smoking, hypertension and diabetes.
  - Encouraging the adoption of healthy lifestyles to minimise the progression of vascular disease.
  - Prescription and monitoring of medication to control risk factors, such as statins or antihypertensives.
- Interdisciplinary collaboration :
  - Teamwork with other specialists, including cardiologists, interventional radiologists and angiologists.
  - Coordination of care with other health professionals, such as vascular nurses, for overall patient monitoring.
- Continuing education and research :
  - Monitoring technological advances and new techniques in vascular surgery.
  - Participation in research to improve treatment methods and patient outcomes.

The importance of vascular surgery in modern medicine is undeniable. These essential clinical roles ensure that vascular surgeons are not only experts in their procedures, but also educators, collaborators and innovators, contributing to the ongoing evolution of the specialty.

The nurse: link between the surgeon, the patient and the team

The operating theatre is a theatre in which each actor plays a vital role. At the centre of this dynamic is the nurse, an essential pivot, acting as the unfailing link between the surgeon, the patient and the entire medical team. This unique position gives nurses a multitude of responsibilities and opportunities to positively influence the patient's care pathway.

- Communication Mediator :
    - The nurse facilitates communication between the patient and the surgeon. They are often the ones who translate complex medical terms into language the patient can understand, while ensuring that the patient's concerns and questions are relayed to the surgeon.
    - Within the team, the nurse coordinates information between the various professionals involved, ensuring that each member is kept informed of relevant updates on the patient's condition.
- Patient Advocate :
    - Nurses ensure that patients' rights are respected, making sure that their wishes and preferences are heard and taken into account.
    - In the event of a complication or misunderstanding, the nurse is often the patient's voice, advocating for their interests and well-being.
- Care Coordinator :
    - Nurses orchestrate a multitude of tasks before, during and after surgery. These range from preparing the patient for the operation to managing post-operative care.

- They work closely with anaesthetists, nursing assistants, technicians and other professionals to ensure that the patient receives consistent, well-coordinated care.
- Educator :
  - The nurse informs the patient and his or her family about what to expect before, during and after surgery. This education may cover post-operative care, pain management or the signs of complications to watch out for.
  - Within the team, nurses can also play a teaching role, sharing their knowledge and expertise with new members or trainees.
- Emotional Support :
  - Surgery can be a stressful experience for the patient. The nurse offers emotional support, reassuring the patient and their family, and providing an empathetic and comforting presence.
  - The nurse also supports the members of the team, offering a listening ear and encouragement during difficult times.
- Resources Manager :
  - The nurse ensures that all the necessary equipment and supplies are available and operational. This may include preparing surgical instruments, managing medicines or coordinating with the pharmacy and other departments.

Nurses are much more than simply carrying out medical orders. They are the guardians of patient safety, the conductors of coordinated care, and the bridge between patient, surgeon and team. In the complex world of vascular surgery, the importance of this role cannot be underestimated.

Stress and emergency management

In the fast-paced world of vascular surgery, where seconds can mean the difference between life and death, the ability to manage stress and respond effectively to emergencies is crucial. Every healthcare professional in vascular surgery, from surgeons to nurses, must master this delicate art to ensure the best possible outcome for the patient.

- Understanding the nature of emergencies :
  - Each emergency situation is unique. It could be a ruptured aneurysm, acute ischaemia or a post-operative complication. Quickly recognising the exact nature of the emergency is the first step to effective intervention.
- Mental and physical preparation :
  - Professionals must be trained to anticipate and react to emergencies. This requires regular simulations, ongoing training and reviews of previous emergencies to ensure that the team is always ready.
- Clear and effective communication:
  - In an emergency situation, every second counts. Clear communication between team members minimises errors and speeds up decision-making.
- Prioritisation :
  - It is essential to assess the situation quickly and determine which actions need to be taken first. This could mean stabilising a patient before moving on to more complex interventions.
- Self-regulation and stress management :
  - Deep breathing techniques, visualisation and even short but regular breaks can help manage stress.

- Recognising your own signs of stress and having strategies for dealing with them is crucial. This can improve not only personal well-being, but also the level of care provided to the patient.
- Post-emergency debriefing :
  - After an emergency situation has been resolved, it is essential to get together with the team to discuss what went well and what could be improved. This not only allows us to learn from each situation, but also to deal with the emotions and stress that can arise after an emergency.
- Emotional support :
  - Emergencies can have a heavy emotional impact on healthcare professionals. It is essential to have support systems in place, whether in the form of discussions with colleagues, counselling or other resources to deal with vicarious trauma and burnout.
- Updating skills and knowledge :
  - Medicine and surgery are constantly evolving. Professionals need to engage in ongoing training to ensure they are up to date with the latest techniques, equipment and procedures.

In the often unpredictable arena of vascular surgery, the ability to manage stress and navigate emergencies competently is not only desirable; it is essential. By cultivating these skills and reinforcing them regularly, professionals can ensure that they offer the best possible level of care to their patients, even in the most adverse circumstances.

Chapter 3:
KNOWLEDGE ABOUT VASCULAR ANATOMY

Circulatory system : an overview

The circulatory system, often referred to as the cardiovascular system, is a marvel of biological engineering, orchestrating the continuous movement of blood through the body, ensuring the transport of oxygen, nutrients, hormones and much more to every cell. Let's take a closer look at this incredible machinery of the human body.

- Heart: the engine of the system
    - Located in the centre of the chest, the heart is a powerful muscle made up of four chambers: two atria and two ventricles. By contracting rhythmically, the heart pumps blood through the body, circulating life within us.
- Blood vessels: the body's highways
    - **Arteries:** These robust channels run from the heart to carry oxygen-rich blood to the body's tissues. The largest of these, the aorta, branches into smaller arteries that serve every region of the body.
    - **Veins:** These vessels carry oxygen-poor blood from the tissues back to the heart. The veins combine to form larger and larger vessels, with the superior vena cava and inferior vena cava carrying blood back to the heart.
    - **Capillaries:** These tiny blood vessels connect the arteries to the veins. Their thin walls allow

exchanges between the blood and the cells, supplying oxygen and nutrients and eliminating waste.
- Blood: the vital mail
  - Made up of red blood cells, white blood cells, platelets and plasma, blood transports oxygen, nutrients, hormones and immune cells to where they are needed. It also plays a crucial role in regulating body temperature, maintaining acid-base balance and protecting against infection.
- Dual circulation: oxygenation and distribution
  - **Pulmonary circulation:** Oxygen-poor blood from the heart is pumped to the lungs via the pulmonary arteries. In the lungs, carbon dioxide is exchanged for fresh oxygen.
  - **Systemic circulation:** Oxygen-rich blood from the lungs is pumped from the heart to the rest of the body via the aorta, nourishing tissues and organs and collecting carbon dioxide and waste products for return to the heart.
- Regulation and maintenance :
  - Complex mechanisms, such as the autonomic nervous system, hormones and pressure receptors, work in harmony to adjust heart rate, force of contraction and blood vessel diameter, ensuring that blood is distributed according to the body's needs.
- Interconnection with other systems :
  - The circulatory system does not operate in a vacuum. It is closely linked to other systems, such as the respiratory system, which oxygenates the blood, the digestive system, which absorbs nutrients, and the excretory system, which eliminates waste.

The circulatory system is truly the crossroads of life, a vital network that ensures that every part of our body receives what it needs to function and that waste products are efficiently eliminated. Without it, life as we know it would be impossible.

Main vessels and their particularities

The circulatory system is a complex web of vessels that carry blood throughout the body. These blood vessels can be broadly classified into arteries, veins and capillaries, but it is useful to look at some of the most important vessels and their distinctive features.

- Arteries
    - **Aorta: This is** the largest and most important artery. It emerges from the left ventricle of the heart and branches into smaller arteries to supply oxygenated blood to the whole body.
    - *Special feature:* Its wall is particularly thick and elastic to withstand the high pressure of the blood ejected by the heart.
    - **Coronary** arteries: These supply the heart itself with oxygen and nutrients.
    - *Special feature:* A blockage here, such as that caused by atherosclerotic plaque, can lead to a heart attack.
    - **Carotid arteries:** These supply the brain with oxygenated blood. They are divided into internal and external carotid arteries.
    - *Special feature:* Occlusion or narrowing of these arteries can increase the risk of stroke.
    - **Pulmonary arteries:** Unlike most arteries, these carry deoxygenated blood from the heart to the lungs for oxygenation.

- *Special feature:* The only arteries to carry oxygen-poor blood.
- Veins
    - **Cava veins:** These are the largest veins in the body and carry deoxygenated blood back to the heart.
    - *Special feature:* They are divided into the superior vena cava (carrying blood from the upper part of the body) and the inferior vena cava (carrying blood from the lower part of the body).
    - **Pulmonary veins:** These carry oxygenated blood from the lungs back to the heart.
    - *Special feature:* Unlike most veins, they carry oxygen-rich blood.
    - **Saphenous veins:** Large superficial veins in the legs.
    - *Particularity:* Frequently involved in varicose veins.
- Capillaries
    - These are the smallest blood vessels, forming networks between arteries and veins.
    - *Special feature:* They have extremely thin walls to allow the exchange of gases, nutrients and waste products between the blood and the tissues.

Each vessel in the circulatory system has a specific structure and function that enable it to meet the body's needs. Understanding these vessels and their particularities is essential to understanding the vast and complex network that sustains life in our bodies.

Common vascular anomalies

Vascular anomalies refer to a wide range of conditions that affect the blood vessels. These conditions may be congenital (present at birth) or acquired during life. Here is an overview of some of the most common vascular anomalies:

- Atherosclerosis :
    - **Description:** Hardening and narrowing of the arteries caused by the accumulation of plaques made up of cholesterol, inflammatory cells and debris.
    - **Consequences:** Can lead to conditions such as coronary heart disease, strokes and peripheral arterial disease.
- Aneurysms :
    - **Description:** abnormal dilation of part of a blood vessel, usually an artery, due to weakness of the vascular wall.
    - **Consequences:** Risk of rupture, which can be fatal, especially in the case of an aortic or cerebral aneurysm.
- Arteriovenous malformations (AVMs) :
    - **Description:** Abnormal connections between arteries and veins, generally present at birth.
    - **Consequences:** May cause bleeding or epileptic seizures if found in the brain.
- Varicose veins :
    - **Description:** Dilated and tortuous veins, generally located in the legs.
    - **Consequences:** Can cause pain, itching, ulcers and other complications.
- Deep vein thrombosis (DVT) :
    - **Description:** Formation of a blood clot in a deep vein, usually in the legs.

- **Consequences:** Risk of pulmonary embolism if the clot travels to the lungs.
- Phlebitis :
  - **Description:** Inflammation of a vein, generally associated with the formation of a blood clot.
  - **Consequences:** May lead to deep vein thrombosis or other complications.
- Arterial stenosis :
  - **Description:** narrowing of an artery due to various causes, including atherosclerosis.
  - **Consequences:** May reduce blood flow to downstream tissues, leading to ischaemia.
- Raynaud's syndrome :
  - **Description:** Temporary narrowing of the small blood vessels in the fingers and toes, usually in response to cold or stress.
  - **Consequences:** Causes whitening or cyanosis of the extremities.
- Vasculitis :
  - **Description:** Inflammation of the walls of blood vessels, which can affect small, medium-sized or large vessels.
  - **Consequences:** Can damage vital organs by reducing their blood supply.

Each vascular anomaly presents unique diagnostic and therapeutic challenges. Prompt and appropriate management is essential to prevent the potentially serious complications associated with these conditions.

Chapter 4:
TECHNIQUES AND STANDARD PROCEDURES

Basics of vascular surgery

Vascular interventions are a set of procedures designed to treat diseases of the blood vessels. These interventions can be surgical, endovascular (using catheters guided inside the vessels) or a combination of the two. Here is an introduction to the basics of these procedures:

- Pre-operative assessment :
    - *Objective:* To determine the extent and location of vascular disease, assess the patient's general condition and identify potential risks.
    - *Common methods:* Doppler, angiography, computed tomography (CT) and magnetic resonance imaging (MRI).
- Anaesthesia :
    - Vascular procedures can be carried out under local, regional or general anaesthetic, depending on the procedure and the surgeon's preference.
- Surgical approaches :
    - *Endarterectomy:* Removal of atherosclerotic plaque from an artery, commonly used to treat carotid stenosis.
    - *Bypass:* Creation of a bypass around a blocked segment of artery using a graft.
    - *Aneurysm repair:* Reinforcement of a dilated aneurysm zone to prevent rupture.
- Endovascular procedures :
    - *Angioplasty: the* use of a balloon to dilate a narrowed or blocked artery.

- *Stent :* Metallic device inserted to keep an artery open after angioplasty.
- *Endoprostheses:* Used to treat aortic aneurysms, these are deployed inside the aneurysm to reinforce it.
- Closing :
  - Small incisions can be closed with sutures, staples or skin adhesive. Larger incisions generally require sutures or staples.
- Post-operative monitoring :
  - *Objective:* Identify and manage potential complications quickly.
  - *Common methods:* Monitoring vital signs, assessing stitches, monitoring blood flow using Doppler, blood tests.
- Rehabilitation and follow-up :
  - Patients may require physiotherapy to regain their mobility.
  - Long-term follow-up is essential to monitor the patency of repaired or treated vessels, and to ensure that the disease does not progress.
- Secondary prevention :
  - Once vascular surgery has been completed, it is crucial to adopt preventive measures to avoid recurrence or progression of the vascular disease.
  - This may include medication (such as anti-platelet drugs), lifestyle changes and regular monitoring.

Understanding the basics of vascular interventions is crucial for healthcare professionals involved in the management of patients with vascular disease. These interventions, when performed correctly and followed by appropriate management, can save lives and improve quality of life.

Assistance during angiography, endarterectomy and other procedures

Nurses play a key role in providing assistance during vascular operations. Whether for angiography, endarterectomy or other procedures, their reassuring presence, technical skills and ability to anticipate the surgeon's needs are essential.

- Angiography :
    - *Preparing the patient:* Explaining the procedure, obtaining consent, checking for allergies (particularly to contrast products), getting the patient settled.
    - *Assistance during the procedure:* Helping to insert the catheter, administering the contrast medium under supervision, monitoring the patient's response, noting observations.
    - *Post-operative care:* Monitor the insertion site for any bleeding or haematomas, monitor vital signs, ensure hydration to eliminate the contrast product.
- Endarterectomy :
    - *Preparing the patient:* Inform the patient of the procedure, check medical history and medication, prepare the skin for the incision.
    - *Assistance during the procedure:* Passing instruments to the surgeon, helping to visualise the operating field, monitoring vital signs and neurological status.
    - *Post-operative care:* Monitoring the incision area, assessing tissue perfusion, monitoring neurological function, managing pain.
- Other interventions :
    - *Bypass:* Assist with graft preparation, monitor anastomosis for bleeding, ensure adequate perfusion of the limb.

- *Stent and angioplasty:* Assist with stent insertion and deployment, administer drugs to prevent clotting, monitor reaction to contrast medium.
- *Aneurysm repair:* Passing instruments, monitoring blood pressure and vital signs, monitoring drains and dressings.

Points common to all interventions :
- **Communication:** Keeping the patient informed throughout the procedure, reassuring in case of anxiety, reporting any anomalies observed to the surgeon or anaesthetist.
- **Sterility:** Ensuring the sterility of the operating field, preventing contamination, ensuring that all instruments are correctly sterilised.
- **Monitoring:** Constantly monitor the patient for signs of distress, allergy or complication.

Effective collaboration between the nurse and the surgeon is essential to ensure the safety and efficacy of vascular interventions. Each member of the team has a unique responsibility, and their synchronisation is crucial for an optimal result.

Post-operative management

The post-operative period is crucial to the patient's recovery and the success of the vascular procedure. The nurse plays a central role in monitoring and caring for the patient during this phase, ensuring that complications are minimised and that the patient is on the road to full recovery.

- Monitoring vital signs :
    - Monitor blood pressure, heart rate, oxygen saturation and temperature.

- Watch for any signs of instability or sudden change.
- Assessment of tissue perfusion :
  - Regularly check the colour, temperature and sensation of the operated limb or area.
  - Assess the distal pulse to ensure there is no circulatory compromise.
- Surgical site monitoring :
  - Examine the incision area regularly for signs of infection, bleeding or oozing.
  - Check that the drains (if present) are working properly and note the quantity and quality of secretions.
- Pain management :
  - Regularly assess the patient's level of pain.
  - Administer analgesics as prescribed and monitor response and side effects.
- Early mobilisation :
  - Encourage the patient to move and walk as soon as it is deemed safe to do so, to prevent complications associated with immobility such as deep vein thrombosis.
- Hydration and nutrition :
  - Monitor fluid intake and output to ensure adequate hydration.
  - Encourage a balanced diet to promote healing.
- Patient education :
  - Instruct the patient on incision care, signs of infection or complications to watch out for.
  - Discuss medication, dosage and possible side effects.
  - Providing information on activity restrictions, returning to work and other day-to-day concerns.

- Planning the outing :
    - Assess the patient's ability to care for themselves at home.
    - Organising follow-up appointments and ensuring that patients have access to all the resources they need for their recovery.
- Communication with the medical team :
    - Working closely with surgeons, anaesthetists and other healthcare professionals to ensure coherent and comprehensive care.
    - Report any concerns or potential complications.

Post-operative management is a combination of clinical assessment, practical nursing care and patient education. It aims to ensure that the patient recovers fully and quickly, while minimising the risk of complications. Effective and careful management during this period can greatly affect long-term patient outcomes.

Chapter 5:
TOOLS AND EQUIPMENT

Introduction to essential tools

In vascular surgery, as in many other areas of medicine, tools play an indispensable role. These instruments, carefully designed and often refined over decades, enable surgeons to perform delicate operations with precision. They are the unfailing allies of healthcare professionals, enabling the human hand to reach, manipulate and repair the sometimes minute structures at the heart of our circulatory system.

When you immerse yourself in the world of vascular surgery, the variety and specialisation of tools can be impressive. The delicate forceps used to manipulate vessels, the probes used to explore them, or the catheters used to introduce other instruments or administer drugs directly into the vascular system, all bear witness to the constant evolution of this medical speciality.

And then there are the more technological tools, such as angiography machines that use X-rays to visualise vessels in real time, or ultrasound to detect blood flow. This high-tech equipment is essential for guiding the surgeon, giving him or her a window onto the hidden world inside our bodies.

But beyond their immediate function, these tools also tell a story. They speak of the challenges that vascular surgery has faced, the innovations that have revolutionised the field, and the constant evolution of knowledge and techniques. Each instrument reflects a need, a clinical situation to be resolved, and they are the fruit of human ingenuity dedicated to saving lives.

So, as a nurse or healthcare professional entering this field, taking the time to understand and respect these tools is crucial. Not only because they are essential to daily practice, but also because they are a symbol of the collective commitment to improving care and the well-being of patients.

Over the next few pages, we'll be exploring these essential tools in depth, but for now let's just salute them: the silent heroes of vascular surgery.

Maintenance, sterilisation and precautions

Vascular surgery, with its delicate procedures and minimal margin for error, demands scrupulous attention not only in terms of technical skill, but also in terms of the maintenance and sterilisation of the tools used. Infection prevention is paramount, and every stage, from preparation through to the operation, must be meticulously orchestrated to guarantee patient safety.

Surgical instruments, from simple forceps to sophisticated electronic devices, are potential vectors of infection if not properly maintained. Sterilisation is an essential step, eliminating all pathogenic micro-organisms that could compromise the success of surgery.

Regular maintenance of equipment ensures that it operates at optimum efficiency. Poorly maintained or faulty tools can not only compromise an operation, but also cause direct harm to the patient. Imaging equipment, for example, must be precisely calibrated to provide clear, accurate images to guide the surgeon during the operation.

But sterilisation is not just about the instruments. The operating environment itself, from the surgical tables to the lights, from the floor to the air, must be rigorously controlled. Strict cleaning and disinfection procedures are put in place, often supervised by dedicated teams who ensure that the operating theatre remains a haven of cleanliness.

In addition to sterilisation, precautions are taken to avoid any other risks. For example, prolonged exposure to the X-rays used in angiography can be harmful. It is therefore essential to limit exposure time and use appropriate protective equipment.

For vascular surgery nurses, this aspect of the profession requires in-depth training. Understanding the nuances of each tool, knowing how and when it should be sterilised, and being aware of the precautions to be taken to protect both the patient and the medical team are all essential skills.

Maintenance, sterilisation and precautions are fundamental pillars of vascular surgery. They reflect a deep commitment to quality of care, safety and clinical excellence, ensuring that every operation is carried out under the best possible conditions.

Modern technology and innovation

Medicine is constantly evolving, and increasingly relies on technological advances to improve diagnosis, treatment and patient care. Vascular surgery is no exception to this trend. The intersection of medical research, biomedical engineering and information technology has led to revolutionary innovations that have transformed this speciality.

The first great revolution was the introduction of advanced medical imaging. Devices such as the angiograph, which uses X-rays to visualise blood vessels in real time, allowed surgeons to accurately diagnose vascular anomalies without the need for invasive surgery. Subsequently, Doppler ultrasound provided a non-invasive window on blood circulation, detecting abnormal or obstructed blood flow with remarkable accuracy.

The digital age has also introduced robotic-assisted surgery. These systems, which are directed by surgeons but benefit from mechanical precision, can perform delicate operations with unrivalled dexterity and accuracy. They also minimise incisions, reducing the risk of infection and speeding up recovery.

Advances in biomaterials have also paved the way for innovations in vascular surgery. For example, stents, small metal or plastic tubes, are used to open narrowed or blocked vessels. These devices, which are constantly being improved, are now designed to be more durable, compatible and sometimes even to administer drugs directly to the site of implantation.

Augmented and virtual reality applications are also gaining ground. They offer surgeons 3D visualisation of vascular structures, enabling more precise surgical planning and better orientation during procedures.

Artificial intelligence and machine learning are also making their way into the field. Sophisticated algorithms can help analyse medical images, detect anomalies and even predict risks based on data models.

However, despite these impressive technological advances, vascular surgery remains fundamentally a profession of humans for humans. Machines can help, but it is the surgeon, with his or her expertise, judgement and compassion, who is at the heart of every successful operation. Modern technology and innovations are tools, extensions of the surgeon's skills, not substitutes. They symbolise the bright future of vascular surgery, combining the best of human ingenuity with the promise of better patient care.

Chapter 6:
INTERACTION WITH THE PATIENT

Pre-operative patient assessment

The pre-operative assessment is a crucial stage in the preparation for surgery. It is the time when the surgeon and his team gather essential information about the patient, assess potential risks and determine the best surgical approach. In vascular surgery, this assessment is all the more crucial because the operations involve structures that supply every nook and cranny of the body with oxygenated blood.

First of all, the patient's medical history is carefully examined. This includes any history of cardiovascular disease, hypertension, diabetes or other conditions that may affect vascular health. Surgeons also look at previous surgical procedures, any medication the patient is currently taking and any family history of vascular disease.

The symptoms presented by the patient are also analysed in depth. Leg pain when walking, wounds that do not heal properly, or signs of poor circulation can all point to a diagnosis.

A series of diagnostic tests is usually ordered. These may include Doppler ultrasound to assess blood flow, angiography to visualise blood vessels, or other imaging tests such as computed tomography (CT) or magnetic resonance imaging (MRI). These tests provide a clear picture of the patient's vascular situation and guide the surgeon in his planning.

Assessment of cardiac function is also essential, as any surgical procedure can put the heart to the test. Tests such as an electrocardiogram (ECG) or echocardiography may be necessary.

The results of laboratory tests, such as blood tests, provide additional information on the patient's general health, coagulation capacity and other parameters that may influence the operation.

From a physical point of view, the patient's mobility, strength and nutritional status can also be assessed. Recovery from surgery can depend in part on these factors.

Finally, the pre-operative assessment also includes a psychological dimension. It is vital to understand the patient's expectations, concerns and emotional state, because surgery, however routine it may be for a surgeon, is often a major event for the patient.

The pre-operative assessment is a multi-dimensional stage that takes into account every aspect of the patient's health and life. It lays the foundations for a successful operation and guides the surgeon and his team through the complex and delicate process of vascular surgery. It is a delicate dance between science, technology and humanity, with the patient's well-being and safety as the ultimate goal.

Educating the patient : explanations and reassurance

The approach of surgery is often a time of anxiety for patients. The unknown, fear of pain, apprehension about possible complications, worries about convalescence... these are all emotions and questions that can overwhelm the patient. In this context, the role of the nurse and the medical team is not just limited to physically preparing the patient for the operation. Education, detailed explanations and reassurance are just as essential.

1. The importance of clear communication :
A well-informed patient is often a more relaxed patient. Explaining in detail the nature of the operation, the key stages of the surgery, and the post-operative course helps to demystify the process. By using clear language, avoiding medical jargon wherever possible, the team can help the patient visualise and understand what to expect.

2. Answering questions :
Each patient is unique and will have his or her own questions and concerns. It is essential to devote time to answering these questions, whether they concern details of the surgery, the length of the hospital stay, possible scarring, or post-operative restrictions.

3. Reassurance about pain and its management :
One of the main concerns is often pain. It is crucial to reassure the patient about pain management, the analgesics that will be administered and alternative methods of pain management.

4. Emphasise the importance of collaboration :
Patients are not simply passive recipients of care. Encouraging them to take an active part in their recovery, whether through breathing or mobility exercises, or simply by complying with medical instructions, means that they play an active role in their own recovery.

5. Value emotional support :
Surgery is not just a physical event. Emotional support, whether in the form of a listening ear, a reassuring presence or links with support groups, can be invaluable.

6. Introducing technology :
With the advent of modern technology, digital tools can also be used to educate patients. Explanatory videos, applications dedicated to surgery or interactive platforms can be used to supplement traditional education.

7. Preparing for the future :
As well as the surgery itself, it is essential to educate patients about the post-operative phase: wound care, rehabilitation, medical follow-up, warning signs to watch out for, etc.

Educating and reassuring a patient before vascular surgery is a multidimensional task that combines technical skill, empathy and communication. It is a stage that, when properly mastered, greatly facilitates the course of the operation and the patient's convalescence. It is a delicate art that combines science and humanity, as each patient's experiences, needs and expectations are unique.

Post-operative follow-up and rehabilitation

The post-operative period in vascular surgery is as essential, if not more so, than the operation itself. It determines the quality of recovery, the minimisation of complications and the achievement of expected results. Rigorous monitoring and appropriate rehabilitation are therefore essential to ensure that patients enjoy the best possible outcome following their operation.

1. The first few hours after the operation :
This is the acute phase, when the patient is closely monitored, often in a recovery room or intensive care unit. The medical team regularly checks vital signs and the condition of the surgical wound, and ensures that there is no bleeding or any other immediate complications.

2. Pain management :
An analgesic protocol is put in place to ensure patient comfort. It is adjusted according to the patient's feedback and the progress of the pain.

3. Vascular monitoring :

The blood flow in the operated area is regularly checked, whether by palpation, auscultation or more sophisticated methods such as Doppler ultrasound.

4. Early mobilisation :

Unless contraindicated, it is advisable to mobilise the patient early on. This promotes better blood circulation, prevents pulmonary complications and stimulates faster recovery.

5. Wound care :

Post-operative care also includes inspecting and cleaning incisions, and checking for infection or wound complications.

6. Education and advice :

Patients are trained in home care, how to recognise the signs of complications, and are given guidelines on physical activity, nutrition and taking medication.

7. Rehabilitation :

Depending on the extent of the operation and the patient's individual needs, a rehabilitation phase may be necessary. This may include physiotherapy, muscle strengthening exercises or education sessions to adopt a healthy lifestyle conducive to vascular health.

8. Long-term follow-up :

Post-operative follow-up does not end when the patient leaves hospital. Regular consultations are scheduled to monitor the patient's progress, adjust treatments and ensure that the results obtained last.

9. Psychological support :

Even successful surgery can have an emotional impact on the patient. Psychological support, whether in the form of individual sessions or support groups, can be beneficial in helping the patient to overcome the emotional challenges of the post-operative period.

10. Integrating technological advances :

With the constant evolution of technology, new tools and methods are regularly added to post-operative monitoring, offering more precise and comfortable ways for patients to monitor their recovery.

Post-operative follow-up in vascular surgery is a comprehensive process, encompassing both medical and psychological aspects. It is a combination of science, humanity and dedication, all with a single objective: the well-being and optimal health of the patient after the operation.

Chapter 7: Complication management

Rapid identification warning signs

In the fast-paced and complex world of vascular surgery, the ability to identify early warning signs can literally mean the difference between life and death. These signs can indicate impending complications, and early recognition allows corrective interventions to be initiated quickly, avoiding potentially serious sequelae.

1. Recognising ischaemia :
Ischaemia refers to a reduction or cessation of blood supply to an organ or tissue. The classic symptoms, particularly for the limbs, are the "5 Ps": Pain, Pallor, Pulselessness, Paresthesia and Paralysis.

2. Monitoring surgical wounds :
Excessive redness, swelling, warmth or purulent discharge may be signs of infection. Separation of the wound edges may indicate a healing problem.

3. Neurological changes :
Sudden changes in consciousness, slurred speech, weakness on one side of the body or changes in vision could indicate a cerebrovascular complication, such as a stroke.

4. Changes in vital signs :
A rapid increase in heart rate, a drop in blood pressure or changes in breathing may be early indicators of internal bleeding or other major complications.

5. Abdominal pain :
Sudden severe abdominal pain after abdominal vascular surgery may signal a complication such as intestinal ischaemia.

6. Oedema :
Sudden swelling of a limb may indicate a blood clot or other vascular obstruction.

7. Skin changes :
Cyanosis (a bluish tinge to the skin) or mottling may be signs of hypoxia or poor perfusion.

8. Respiratory symptoms :
Shortness of breath, sudden chest pain or coughing up bloody sputum may indicate pulmonary complications such as embolism.

9. Varicose veins or swollen veins :
The sudden appearance of dilated veins or swollen areas may suggest venous obstruction or thrombosis.

10. Unexplained pain :
Any sudden, severe pain with no obvious cause after vascular surgery should be taken seriously and assessed immediately.

In vascular care, careful monitoring and early identification of warning signs are essential. These sometimes subtle clinical clues are warning signs that something is wrong. Prompt and appropriate action on these signs can prevent major complications, improving patient outcomes.

Emergency and response protocols

Vascular surgery, which focuses on the management of blood vessels, is naturally prone to emergency situations. Emergency and intervention protocols are used to guide the medical team through the essential steps for responding quickly and effectively to these crises, while maximising patient safety.

1. Initial assessment :
   - **Vital stabilisation:** Prioritising ABC (Airway, Breathing, Circulation).

- **Rapid assessment:** Identify the main problem, note vital signs and assess neurological status.
- **Communication:** Immediately notify the vascular surgeon or specialist on call.

2. Acute arterial thrombosis :
   - **Recognition:** Quickly identify the "5 Ps" (Pain, Pallor, Pulselessness, Paresthesia, Paralysis).
   - **Intervention:** Initiate anticoagulation, prepare the patient for possible emergency surgery to restore blood flow.

3. Aneurysm rupture :
   - **Recognition:** Intense abdominal or back pain, drop in blood pressure, pulsatile mass.
   - **Intervention:** haemodynamic stabilisation, rapid preparation for surgical or endovascular intervention.

4. Pulmonary embolism :
   - **Recognition:** Dyspnoea, chest pain, syncope.
   - **Intervention:** Stabilisation, anticoagulation, cardiac ultrasound or chest CT scan depending on the situation.

5. Mesenteric ischaemia :
   - **Recognition:** Abdominal pain disproportionate to the clinical examination, lactic acidosis.
   - **Intervention:** resuscitation, anticoagulation, surgical or endovascular intervention to restore perfusion.

6. Post-operative complications :
   - **Haemorrhage:** Monitoring drains, vital signs and dressings.
   - **Graft thrombosis:** Monitor distal pulse and irrigated area.
   - **Infections:** Identify early signs such as fever, redness or discharge.

7. Complications associated with vascular access :
   - **Haematoma:** Compression, monitoring and ultrasound if necessary.
   - **Infection:** removal of catheter, culture and initiation of antibiotics.

8. Installation of specific equipment :
Some equipment, such as circulatory assistance pumps, require specific protocols in the event of malfunction or complications.
9. Transfer and transport :
Have protocols for the safe transfer of patients between departments, or to specialist centres for more in-depth treatment.
10. Training and simulations :
Organise regular emergency simulations to ensure that the whole team is familiar with the protocols and able to intervene quickly if necessary.

Preparation and rapid intervention are the watchwords when it comes to vascular surgery emergencies. Standardised and regularly updated protocols ensure that, faced with any critical situation, the medical team knows exactly how to act to guarantee the best possible outcome for the patient.

Emotional support for patients and the family

Vascular surgery, like other medical interventions, can be a source of intense stress not only for the patient, but also for his or her family. The anticipation of surgery, the fear of complications, and the general unknown of the medical process can be overwhelming. The role of medical staff is not just limited to the technicalities of medicine, but also encompasses emotional support for the patient and their family.

1. The importance of listening :
The first step in emotional support is to actively listen to the concerns of the patient and their family. This enables

fears and apprehensions to be identified and responded to appropriately.

2. Clear and transparent information :
- **Pre-operative explanations:** Explain the procedure, its importance, expected benefits and potential risks.
- **Post-operative update:** Information on the progress of the operation, the results and the next steps.

3. Availability and presence :
Staff who are accessible to answer questions or simply to be there when patients or their families need to talk are essential.

4. Encourage visits :
The presence of loved ones can be a powerful remedy for anxiety. Encouraging visits within the limits of hospital protocols can be beneficial for the patient's emotional well-being.

5. Training teams in empathic communication :
Staff must be trained to communicate empathically, showing understanding and compassion, without minimising the patient's concerns.

6. Rest areas for families :
Dedicated spaces where families can rest, recharge their batteries and enjoy a moment of tranquillity are essential.

7. Involve specialists if necessary :
Psychologists, social workers or spiritual care counsellors can provide specialist support depending on individual needs.

8. Support groups :
Support groups for patients and families going through similar experiences can be a source of comfort and encouragement.

9. Respect for culture and beliefs :
Recognising and respecting the cultural and religious beliefs of patients and their families is crucial to providing them with appropriate support.

10. Preparing to return home :
Explain post-operative care and warning signs in detail, and provide resources for emotional support after discharge.

11. Feedback :
After discharge, a follow-up appointment to assess the patient's medical condition and to discuss any emotional issues may be beneficial.

Surgery is not just a physical experience. It profoundly affects the mind and emotions of patients and those around them. Integrating emotional support into the care process not only promotes physical healing, but also the psychological well-being of all those involved.

Chapter 8:
INTERPROFESSIONAL COMMUNICATION

Working with surgeons, anaesthetists and technicians

The world of vascular surgery is interdisciplinary by nature. Successful procedures, from diagnosis to treatment, depend on harmonious collaboration between different healthcare professionals. This dynamic interaction, far from being mere professional coexistence, is the very essence of optimal patient care.

1. Team dynamics :
Each member, from the surgeon to the anaesthetist, the nurse and the technician, brings a unique expertise to the table. This professional complementarity is the foundation of safe and effective care.

2. Pre-operative preparation :
- **With the surgeon:** The nurse works together to prepare the patient, to ensure that all the necessary investigations have been carried out, and that the patient has been properly informed.
- **With the anaesthetist:** A pre-anaesthetic assessment is crucial to anticipate risks and ensure optimal sedation or anaesthesia.

3. During the operation :
- **Synchronisation with the surgeon:** The nurse provides the necessary instruments, anticipates the stages of the surgery, and can help manage emergencies.
- **Interaction with the anaesthetist:** Monitoring the patient's well-being, communicating fluid, medication or transfusion requirements.

- **With the technician:** Ensuring that the equipment is functional, sterile and available.

4. Post-operative :
The nurse acts as a bridge between the sleeping or semi-conscious patient and the specialists, guaranteeing continuity of care and monitoring.

5. Protocols and procedures :
Standardised procedures, clearly understandable and accepted by all, encourage smooth collaboration.

6. Regular meetings and training :
Periodic meetings to discuss cases, share feedback, or even take part in joint training courses strengthen team cohesion.

7. Open communication :
An environment where each member feels free to express their concerns, suggestions or questions is essential to avoid errors and ensure optimal care.

8. Mutual respect :
The traditional medical hierarchy is evolving towards a more team-centred approach. Recognising and valuing the contribution of each member, whatever their title, is crucial.

9. Emergency scenarios :
In critical moments, efficient collaboration between all those involved is vital. Emergency simulations can be set up to train the team to work together in these situations.

10. Constructive feedback :
The possibility of feedback, whether positive or negative, allows each member of the team to continually improve.

Collaboration in vascular surgery is not a luxury, but a necessity. It ensures that patients receive the best possible care by mobilising collective expertise in a perfectly synchronised dance of concerted effort.

Sharing information with paramedics

Sharing information with the paramedical team is an essential pillar of care in vascular surgery. Paramedics, including nurses, laboratory technicians, care assistants and other specialists, play a major role in the continuum of care. Effective communication with them ensures patient safety, the effectiveness of interventions and the overall well-being of the patient.

1. Importance of transmitting information :
Omitted, incomplete or incorrect information can lead to medical errors, delays in treatment or poor coordination.

2. Medical records and reports :
Regular updating of medical records, observations and reports ensures that everyone involved has access to the most up-to-date information about the patient.

3. Daily briefings :
Handover meetings, often held at shift changeover, are used to update the team on the condition of patients, planned interventions and any special concerns.

4. Communication tools :
The use of digital tools, such as hospital information systems, can facilitate the real-time sharing of relevant information.

5. Training and education :
Organise training sessions for paramedics on the specifics of vascular surgery, the warning signs and essential procedures.

6. Clear protocols :
Implementing standardised protocols for common situations ensures that everyone involved knows how to act consistently.

7. Feedback from paramedics :
Encouraging the paramedical team to provide feedback, ask questions and share their observations can improve the quality of care and strengthen collaboration.

8. Coordination with specialists :
Vascular surgery often requires the involvement of other specialities (radiology, cardiology, etc.). Ensuring that paramedics are informed of the recommendations or interventions of these specialists is essential.

9. Preparing for the operation :
Providing details of the type of operation, the patient's specific needs and any complications means that paramedics can prepare the operating environment appropriately.

10. Emergency management :
Establish clear communication protocols in the event of an emergency to ensure a rapid and coordinated response.

11. Confidentiality :
All information shared must respect patient confidentiality and must only be passed on to healthcare professionals directly involved in the patient's care.

Effective, transparent communication with paramedics is crucial to ensuring holistic management in vascular surgery. It not only enhances the quality of care, but also builds trust and collaboration between the various parties involved.

Navigating situations difficult communication

Vascular surgery, like other medical specialities, can present delicate communication situations. Whether it's announcing an unexpected diagnosis, managing the expectations of an anxious patient or resolving conflicts within the team, it's vital to know how to navigate with tact and empathy.

1. Recognising the difficulty :
The first step is to recognise that a situation is complex. Whether it's a misunderstanding, bad news or tension in the team, awareness is the first step towards resolution.

2. Active listening :
Lending an attentive ear not only helps to understand the source of the problem, but also shows the other party that their concerns are being taken seriously.

3. Empathy and compassion :
Putting yourself in the other person's shoes, whether it's a patient, a family member or a colleague, helps you to formulate more sensitive and appropriate responses.

4. Clarification :
If the source of the difficulty is a misunderstanding, it is essential to ask for clarification. Ask open-ended questions to get a clearer picture of the situation.

5. Simple language :
Particularly in the medical field, it is crucial to ensure that the patient and their family understand the information. Avoid medical jargon and make sure your explanations are clear.

6. Managing your emotions :
It's natural to experience emotions in tense situations. However, it is essential to recognise and manage them so that they do not get in the way of communication.

7. Asking for help :
In certain situations, it can be beneficial to call on a mediator, whether a colleague, a supervisor or even a professional trained in mediation.

8. Offering solutions :
Rather than focusing solely on the problem, try to work together to find solutions. This can help divert attention from negative emotions and steer the conversation towards a positive outcome.

9. Taking a step back :
If a situation becomes too tense, it can be useful to take a break. This allows you to regain your composure, think about the best way to proceed and approach the situation with a refreshed perspective.

10. Training and education :
Consider taking training courses in communication, conflict resolution or counselling to improve your communication skills in difficult situations.

Every difficult communication situation is unique, and there is no one-size-fits-all solution. However, by adopting an empathetic, thoughtful and proactive approach, it is possible to successfully navigate most of these situations, to the benefit of the patient, the team and the carer themselves.

Chapter 9:
UPDATE AND TECHNOLOGICAL INNOVATIONS

Latest advances in vascular imaging

Vascular imaging is a constantly evolving field, propelled by technological advances and scientific innovations. These recent developments aim to improve diagnostic accuracy, reduce the invasiveness of procedures and increase patient safety. Here are some of the major advances in this field:

- **Computed tomography angiography (Angio-CT)**: Although Angio-CT is not new, recent improvements in algorithms and machines have made it possible to obtain higher resolution images while reducing the radiation dose to patients.
- **Magnetic resonance angiography (MRA)**: MRA, which uses magnetic waves rather than X-rays, has seen significant improvements in terms of the speed and clarity of images. It is particularly useful for patients where exposure to radiation needs to be minimised.
- **Optical coherence imaging (OCT)**: This technique provides microscopic images of the vessels, enabling abnormalities to be detected at a very early stage or delicate operations to be guided.
- **Image fusion techniques**: By combining different imaging modalities (e.g. ultrasound and fluoroscopy), these techniques provide a complete and detailed view of the area of interest, helping clinicians with guided interventions.
- **Elastography**: This technique measures tissue stiffness, providing valuable information about vascular health and the potential risk of aneurysm.

- **Molecular imaging**: This is an exciting frontier of research that aims to visualise specific molecular processes inside vessels, enabling early detection of vascular disease at a molecular level.
- **Radiation reduction technology** : The new imaging systems are equipped with advanced technologies that minimise the radiation dose received by patients while maintaining image quality.
- **Advanced analysis software**: Thanks to artificial intelligence and machine learning, software can now help to automatically detect anomalies, estimate blood flow or even predict the risk of certain vascular pathologies.
- **Three-dimensional (3D) imaging techniques and augmented reality**: These techniques provide a three-dimensional view of vascular structures, making it easier to plan and carry out interventions.
- **Micro-cameras and vascular endoscopy**: Small devices capable of navigating vessels and providing a detailed internal view, useful for targeted interventions.

These advances, while fascinating, are only the tip of the iceberg. The field of vascular imaging continues to evolve, promising even more accurate, faster and less invasive techniques for patients. For those working in the medical sector, it is crucial to keep abreast of new techniques and technologies in order to provide the best possible care.

Simulations and virtual training for nurses

In the age of digitalisation and advanced technologies, nursing education has evolved considerably. Simulations and virtual training have emerged as essential tools for providing practical education without the risks associated with real clinical situations. Let's take a look at how these methods are revolutionising nursing education.

1. Advantages of simulations :
   - **Risk-free learning:** Students can practise complex procedures or manage emergencies without putting real patients at risk.
   - **Repetition:** Simulations allow you to repeat a procedure as many times as necessary, encouraging mastery and confidence.
   - **Immediate feedback:** Simulation systems often offer real-time feedback, enabling students to correct mistakes on the spot.
2. Types of simulation :
   - **High-fidelity mannequins:** These mannequins faithfully reproduce human physiological reactions, providing a realistic experience of patient care.
   - **Virtual reality-based simulations:** Using VR goggles, students can immerse themselves in a virtual hospital environment, practising skills and interacting with virtual patients.
   - **Serious games and educational applications:** Games designed for training purposes enable learning while having fun, boosting student engagement.
3. Virtual training :
   - **Online learning platforms:** courses, modules and workshops can be accessed anywhere at any time, offering students flexibility.
   - **Webinars and virtual conferences:** experts in the field can share their knowledge with students from all over the world, breaking down geographical barriers.
   - **Augmented reality:** By superimposing digital information on the real environment, it offers an enriched learning experience.

4. Evaluation and feedback :
- **Video recordings:** Simulation sessions can be recorded and viewed for detailed evaluation.
- **Artificial intelligence:** Some advanced systems use AI to provide accurate, personalised feedback on student performance.

5. Challenges and considerations :
- **Cost:** The initial investment in simulation technology can be high, although the long-term benefits often justify the cost.
- **Training the trainers:** To maximise the effectiveness of the simulations, the teachers themselves need to be trained to use these tools.
- **A complement, not a substitute:** While simulations offer enormous advantages, they should not entirely replace real clinical experience.

Simulations and virtual training enrich nursing education, providing hands-on experience in a controlled environment. By integrating these modern tools with traditional teaching methods, we can prepare the next generation of nurses to deliver outstanding care in a constantly changing medical world.

Telesurgery and telemedicine in vascular surgery

Telesurgery and telemedicine represent a fusion of medical technology and information technology, opening up new horizons for patient care. In the field of vascular surgery, these advances promise to improve access to care, the precision of operations and the training of professionals.

1. Telesurgery :
- **Definition:** Telesurgery refers to the remote performance of surgical procedures using robots

controlled by surgeons via a secure Internet connection.
- Advantages :
  - **Extended access:** Enables patients in remote areas to have access to specialist surgeons.
  - **Greater precision:** Surgical robots can perform extremely precise movements, reducing the risk of errors.
  - **Reduced surgeon fatigue:** Prolonged operations can be less exhausting when the surgeon controls a robot.
- Challenges :
  - **Dependence on technology:** Any technological malfunction can pose a risk.
  - **Training:** Surgeons must be trained to use these systems.
  - **Costs:** The initial investment in robotic equipment is high.

2. Telemedicine in vascular surgery :
   - **Remote consultations:** Vascular surgeons can assess, diagnose and advise patients located at a distance using videoconferencing platforms.
   - **Post-operative monitoring:** Telemedicine makes it possible to monitor patients after an operation, assess healing and detect any complications without the need for frequent travel.
   - **Medical collaboration:** Surgeons can work with other specialists remotely to discuss complex cases and draw up treatment plans.
   - **Education and training:** Telemedicine also offers continuing education opportunities for surgeons and medical teams.

3. Future implications :
   - **Expanding access:** With the democratisation of technology, more and more patients around the world could have access to specialist care.

- **Technological innovations:** Future advances could include improved haptics for telesurgery, augmented reality for visualising blood vessels and artificial intelligence for diagnostic assistance.
- **Standards and regulations** : As these technologies become more widespread, it will be essential to establish standards to guarantee patient safety.

Telesurgery and telemedicine in vascular surgery represent a promising fusion of technology and medicine. As these methods continue to develop, they have the potential to transform the way care is delivered, making vascular surgery more accessible and more accurate for patients around the world.

Chapter 10: RISK MANAGEMENT AND PATIENT SAFETY

Identifying and anticipating potential hazards

While vascular surgery is an essential part of modern medicine, it also has its share of potential hazards. Identifying and anticipating these risks is crucial to ensuring patient safety and smooth operations.

1. Hazard identification :
   - **Haemorrhage:** An ever-present risk in surgery, especially when operating on blood vessels. Uncontrolled haemorrhage can have serious consequences.
   - **Thrombosis and embolism:** Blood clots can form following surgery, potentially blocking vital blood vessels.
   - **Infections:** Any surgical procedure exposes the patient to a risk of infection, whether local (at the incision site) or systemic.
   - **Nerve damage:** Nerves close to the operation sites may be damaged, leading to pain, numbness or loss of function.
   - **Anaesthetic complications:** Adverse reactions to anaesthesia may include allergies, respiratory problems or effects on the cardiovascular system.
   - **Graft or stent failure:** When foreign materials, such as stents, are introduced into the body, there is a risk of rejection or failure.
2. Anticipation and prevention :
   - **Detailed pre-operative assessment:** A thorough assessment of the patient, including their medical

history, previous surgery and particular risks, is essential.
- **Meticulous surgical planning:** Precise planning of the operation, with high-quality images and vessel mapping, means there are fewer surprises during surgery.
- **Atraumatic techniques:** Use of instruments and techniques that minimise trauma to tissues and vessels.
- **Prophylactic antibiotics:** In some cases, administering antibiotics before the operation can reduce the risk of infection.
- **Post-operative monitoring:** Close observation after the operation enables any complications to be detected and treated quickly.
- **Ongoing training:** Ensuring that surgeons and the medical team are regularly trained in the latest techniques, technologies and safety protocols.
- **Emergency preparedness:** Have clear protocols in place in the event of an emergency, such as haemorrhage, and ensure that the whole team is trained to implement them.

Whilst recognising that vascular surgery, like any medical procedure, carries risks, rigorous preparation, in-depth knowledge and careful monitoring can go a long way towards minimising these dangers.

Safety protocols and checklists

Safety protocols and checklists are essential for ensuring the safety of patients and healthcare professionals in vascular surgery. They serve to standardise procedures, minimise omissions and ensure a consistent approach to each operation.

1. Before the operation :
   - Preoperative assessment :
     - Collect the patient's medical history.
     - Conducting a physical examination.
     - Carry out relevant laboratory tests (e.g. coagulation tests).
     - Check for a history of allergies, particularly to anaesthetics or specific drugs.
     - Assess the need for antibiotic prophylaxis.
   - Informed consent :
     - Ensure that the patient has been informed of the risks, benefits and alternatives of the operation.
     - Obtain and document signed informed consent.
   - Preparation of the surgical site :
     - Shaving if necessary.
     - Cleaning and disinfecting the site.
2. During the operation :
   - Operating theatre safety checklist (based on WHO protocol) :
     - Before inducing anaesthesia: Check the patient's identity, the type of operation planned and the surgical site.
     - Before the skin incision: Confirm all the details of the operation, make sure the team is ready, and confirm that all the necessary equipment is present and working.
     - Before the patient leaves the operating theatre: check the integrity of the sutures, count the instruments and compresses, note any complications, and discuss post-operative recommendations.
   - Anaesthetic management :
     - Continuous monitoring of vital signs.
     - Administration and monitoring of anaesthetic drugs.

- Make sure the patient is well oxygenated and ventilated.
3. After the operation :
  - Post-operative monitoring :
    - Monitor vital signs.
    - Assess pain and administer analgesics if necessary.
    - Monitor bleeding or other secretions at the surgical site.
    - Assess distal vascular function (pulse, colour, temperature).
  - Wound care :
    - Check the wound regularly for any signs of infection.
    - Change dressings as instructed or if soiled.
  - Debriefing with the team:
    - Discuss any problems or complications that have arisen during the operation.
    - Review what went well and identify areas for improvement.

These protocols and checklists are just an example of what can be used in vascular surgery. It is essential that each medical establishment adapts these lists to its specific needs, the procedures performed and the resources available. Regular training and updates are also crucial to ensure that all staff are aware of best practice and safety procedures.

The role of the nurse in improving the quality of care

Nurses play a central and indispensable role in providing and improving patient care. Their unique position at the crossroads of interactions between doctors, patients, families and other healthcare professionals means they can make a significant contribution to the quality of care. Here is a detailed exploration of this vital role.

1. Ongoing assessment of the patient's needs :
   - Thanks to their constant presence with patients, the nurses regularly assess their condition, noting any changes in their physical or psychological state.
   - This ongoing assessment enables us to anticipate and respond rapidly to patients' changing needs.
2. Promoting patient safety :
   - Nurses ensure patient safety, for example by making sure that medication is administered correctly and that the risk of falls is minimised.
   - They are often the first to notice and point out potential errors or anomalies in the care process.
3. Care coordination :
   - Nurses coordinate the work of the various healthcare professionals involved in a patient's care, ensuring a harmonious multidisciplinary approach.

4. Patient and family education :
   - Informing patients and their families about illnesses, treatments, post-operative care and prevention is a key function of nurses.
   - This education helps to improve adherence to treatment and to empower patients to take responsibility for managing their own health.
5. Advocacy for patient needs :
   - Nurses defend the interests and needs of patients, ensuring that their voices are heard and their rights respected.
6. Participation in clinical research :
   - Many nurses are involved in research, contributing to the improvement of evidence-based practice and innovation in care.

7. Contribution to training and mentoring :
    - Experienced nurses play an essential role in training and guiding new generations of nurses, ensuring that best practice is continually passed on.
8. Process improvement :
    - Thanks to their day-to-day experience, nurses often identify areas for improvement in care protocols and processes, and can play an active part in optimising them.
9. Communication and collaboration :
    - Nurses promote open communication between patients, families and medical teams, ensuring that all stakeholders are informed and involved in the care process.
10. Emotional support :
    - In addition to physical care, nurses provide psychological and emotional support to patients and their families, reinforcing the human dimension of care.

The role of the nurse goes far beyond simply providing technical care. He or she is a central pillar of quality care, guaranteeing not only the safety and well-being of patients, but also the efficiency and humanity of the healthcare system as a whole.

Chapter 11:
PHARMACOLOGY IN VASCULAR SURGERY

Commonly used medicines and their mechanism of action

Medicines are compounds designed to treat, prevent or diagnose disease. They have different mechanisms of action that determine how they work in the body. Here is a list of some commonly used classes of drugs and their mechanism of action:

- Antibiotics (such as penicillin) :
    - Mechanism: They kill or inhibit the growth of bacteria. Some work by disrupting the bacteria's cell wall, while others inhibit their ability to synthesise proteins or copy their DNA.
- Non-steroidal anti-inflammatory drugs (NSAIDs such as ibuprofen):
    - Mechanism: They inhibit the enzymes (mainly cyclooxygenase) responsible for producing prostaglandins, molecules which play a role in inflammation and pain.
- Statins (such as atorvastatin) :
    - Mechanism: They inhibit an enzyme (HMG-CoA reductase) required for the production of cholesterol by the liver, thereby reducing blood cholesterol levels.
- Anticoagulants (such as warfarin) :
    - Mechanism: They prevent blood clotting by interfering with the coagulation cascade or other blood factors.

- Antivirals (such as oseltamivir) :
  - Mechanism: They inhibit the ability of viruses to enter cells, replicate or assemble and release new viral particles.
- Antihypertensives (such as beta-blockers) :
  - Mechanism: They act by relaxing blood vessels, reducing blood volume or decreasing the force and speed of cardiac contraction, thereby lowering blood pressure.
- Antidiabetics (such as metformin) :
  - Mechanism: They increase insulin sensitivity, stimulate insulin release or reduce glucose production by the liver.
- Antipsychotics (such as risperidone) :
  - Mechanism: They modulate the activity of certain neurotransmitters in the brain, in particular dopamine and serotonin.
- Antidepressants (such as selective serotonin reuptake inhibitors, SSRIs):
  - Mechanism: They increase the availability of certain neurotransmitters in the brain, mainly serotonin, by inhibiting their reuptake into synapses.
- Opiates (such as morphine) :
- Mechanism: They act on opioid receptors in the brain to reduce the perception of pain.

This list is far from exhaustive, as there are thousands of medicines, each with its own mechanism of action. Before taking any medicine, it is always essential to consult a healthcare professional to understand its effects, its mechanism of action and any interactions with other medicines.

Drug interactions and side effects

When several medicines are taken simultaneously, they may interact with each other in predictable or unpredictable ways. These interactions may affect the effectiveness of the medicines or increase the risk of side effects.

Drug interactions :
- Pharmacodynamic interactions :
  - They occur when two drugs have similar or opposite effects on the same physiological function. For example, taking an antihypertensive with a drug that raises blood pressure.
- Pharmacokinetic interactions :
  - These interactions modify the absorption, distribution, metabolism or excretion of a drug. For example, some drugs can inhibit or induce liver enzymes that metabolise other drugs, thereby altering their blood levels.
- Food interactions :
  - Certain foods can interfere with the absorption or metabolism of medicines. For example, grapefruit can increase the levels of certain drugs in the blood by inhibiting an enzyme involved in their metabolism.
- Interactions with supplements or medicinal plants :
  - Products such as St John's Wort can interact with drugs such as antidepressants or anticoagulants, altering their effectiveness or increasing the risk of side effects.

Side effects:
- Common side effects:
  - These effects are generally benign and predictable. For example, drowsiness caused

by antihistamines or constipation caused by certain opioids.
- Serious side effects :
  - These are rare but potentially dangerous effects, such as severe allergic reactions or heart problems induced by certain drugs.
- Delayed side effects :
  - They can appear long after the start of treatment, like certain side effects of chemotherapy.
- Dose-related side effects :
  - Some effects are directly linked to the dose of medicine administered. For example, an overdose of aspirin can cause hearing problems.
- Idiosyncratic side effects :
  - These are unpredictable reactions that are not dose-related and are not necessarily explained by the known pharmacological properties of the drug.

Drug interactions and side effects are two major concerns when prescribing and taking medicines. Open communication between patient and healthcare professional, thorough knowledge of medicines and regular monitoring can help minimise the associated risks and ensure safe and effective drug therapy.

Post-operative pain management

Post-operative pain is a common concern for patients and medical staff alike. It can affect recovery, length of hospitalisation and increase the risk of complications. Effective management of postoperative pain is essential to optimise patient recovery and improve patient comfort.

Pain assessment :
The first step in pain management is pain assessment. Visual or verbal pain scales, such as the Visual Analogue Scale, can help quantify the level of pain felt by the patient.
Pharmacological approaches :

- Non-opioid analgesics :
  - For example, paracetamol or non-steroidal anti-inflammatory drugs (NSAIDs) such as ibuprofen. These drugs are often used for mild to moderate pain.
- Opiates :
  - For moderate to severe pain, drugs such as morphine, oxycodone or tramadol may be prescribed. They are effective, but can have side effects such as constipation, drowsiness and the risk of dependence.
- Additives :
  - Certain drugs, such as tricyclic antidepressants or anticonvulsants, can be used to reinforce the analgesic effect or treat specific types of pain, such as neuropathic pain.

Non-pharmacological approaches :
- Relaxation techniques :
  - Deep breathing, meditation or visualisation can help reduce the perception of pain.
- Thermotherapy and cryotherapy :
  - Applying heat or cold may provide temporary relief.
- Transcutaneous electrical nerve stimulation (TENS) :
  - It uses electrical currents to relieve pain.
- Physiotherapy :
  - Movement and exercise can help reduce pain and improve function.

Patient-centred strategies :
- Patient education :
    - Inform patients about what they can expect in terms of pain, the treatment options available, and the importance of communicating their pain levels.
- Personalised care plan :
    - Every patient is unique. Their pain management plan must be adapted to their needs, preferences and overall state of health.

Managing postoperative pain is a crucial aspect of care after surgery. It requires a multi-dimensional approach that combines pharmacological and non-pharmacological methods, with an emphasis on listening to patients and their needs. Effective management can greatly improve patient satisfaction and promote rapid, uncomplicated recovery.

Chapter 12:
SPECIFIC ETHICAL CHALLENGES VASCULAR SURGERY

Allocation of resources and patient prioritisation

In a medical environment, every decision is of particular importance, especially when it comes to allocating limited resources and prioritising patients. In vascular surgery, this task is further complicated by the urgent and sometimes unpredictable nature of the cases, as well as the complexity of the interventions.

Understanding what's at stake :
Resources, whether material, human or financial, are often limited. Optimum use of these resources is vital if we are to guarantee quality care for all patients. Prioritisation therefore becomes an essential tool for determining who should be treated first, based on severity, urgency and the chances of success of the intervention.

Resource allocation methods :
- Needs assessment :
    - A regular inventory of equipment, staff, medicines and other resources enables current and future needs to be identified.
- Equipment optimisation :
    - Regular maintenance, ongoing staff training on the optimum use of equipment and periodic technological updates.
- Personnel management :
    - Ensuring a balanced distribution of tasks, offering ongoing training and ensuring the well-

being of team members to maximise their efficiency.

Patient prioritisation criteria :
- Medical emergencies :
  - Patients with an immediate life-threatening condition, such as a ruptured aneurysm, are naturally treated as a priority.
- Expected clinical benefit :
  - Prioritise interventions that offer a significant benefit in terms of survival or quality of life.
- Waiting :
  - Take into account the patient's waiting time, especially in the case of elective surgery.
- Age and co-morbidities :
  - Although age should not be a discriminatory criterion, it can be taken into account in combination with other factors, such as co-morbidities, to assess the chances of post-operative success.

Ethical challenges :

Prioritisation can sometimes lead to ethical dilemmas, particularly when a choice has to be made between two patients presenting a similar emergency. It is essential to have clear, fair and transparent guidelines to guide these decisions.

Allocating resources and prioritising patients in vascular surgery are ongoing challenges that require strategic, ethical and patient-centred thinking. Close collaboration between surgeons, nurses, administrators and other members of the medical team is essential to ensure optimal care for all patients, despite resource constraints.

Refusal of treatment and patient autonomy

Patient autonomy is a fundamental pillar of modern medicine. It reflects respect for individual rights, enabling each person to play an active role in decisions concerning their health. However, in vascular surgery, as in other medical disciplines, a patient's refusal of treatment can pose ethical and practical challenges for healthcare professionals.

The importance of patient autonomy :
Autonomy is based on the idea that each individual has the right to make decisions about his or her own body. It is a recognition of the right to freedom and human dignity. In medicine, this means that the patient has the right to refuse treatment, even if it may be contrary to his or her well-being.

Common reasons for refusing treatment :
- **Religious or cultural beliefs:** Some patients refuse procedures because of their personal beliefs.
- **Fear of complications:** Fears about the risks of surgery or side effects can deter some patients.
- **Misunderstanding:** An insufficient or misunderstood explanation of the need for or benefits of an intervention can lead to refusal.
- **Past experiences:** Previous treatments that have gone wrong can have a negative influence on the patient's decision.

Navigating through treatment refusal :
- **Open communication:** Establish a dialogue with the patient to understand the reason for their refusal and address their concerns.
- **Education:** Providing clear, precise and comprehensible information on the proposed treatment, its benefits and risks.

- **Involving the family:** In certain cultures or situations, discussions with the family can help to clarify the patient's decision.
- **Consider alternatives:** If possible, propose alternatives that might be more acceptable to the patient.
- **Informed consent:** Ensuring that the patient fully understands the consequences of refusal.

Ethical aspects :

Although healthcare professionals have a duty to protect the health and well-being of their patients, they must also respect patient autonomy. This can create conflict, especially if the patient refuses treatment that could save their life or significantly improve their quality of life.

Refusal of treatment is a complex challenge in vascular surgery. Although it can be difficult to accept such a decision, respect for patient autonomy is essential. Through open communication, patient-centred education and an empathetic approach, healthcare professionals can help patients make informed decisions that truly reflect their wishes and values.

End of life and vascular surgery

When it comes to vascular surgery, the stakes can be immense. Interventions designed to improve circulation, prevent strokes or treat aneurysms can be life-saving, but they can also be risky, particularly for elderly patients or those in the advanced stages of a disease. In this context, how do we manage the end of life? How do we balance the hope of improvement with the reality of possible risks and complications?

Vascular surgery in old age :
Advancing age can bring with it a host of co-morbidities, sometimes making surgery more risky. However, advances in techniques and knowledge mean that we can now offer elderly patients operations that were previously considered too risky.

Consider the benefits and risks:
- **Post-operative quality of life:** Will the operation significantly improve the patient's quality of life, or could it deteriorate it further, especially in the event of complications?
- **Estimated lifespan:** Is the operation justified if the patient only has a few months or years to live?

Ethical challenges :
- **Patient autonomy:** Patients have the right to choose or refuse treatment, even in the face of a potential end of life. Informing them correctly is essential.
- **Non-maleficence:** Health professionals must avoid causing harm. Is a risky intervention justified?
- **Beneficence:** Carers must act in the patient's best interests, balancing benefits and risks.

Advance directives and care planning :

When a patient is terminally ill or facing a risky surgical decision, it is essential to discuss the patient's wishes regarding his or her end of life, and to draw up advance directives if this has not already been done.

The role of the medical team :
- **Communication:** Openly discuss the benefits, risks and alternatives available.
- **Support:** Offering emotional support to the patient and their family, and guiding them through these difficult decisions.

- **Interdisciplinarity:** Working with other healthcare professionals, such as palliative care specialists, to ensure a comprehensive approach.

The end of life in vascular surgery poses major challenges, both medical and ethical. As healthcare professionals, it is essential to support patients and their families with empathy, honesty and expertise, while respecting their choices and values. By doing so, we can hope to offer a dignified end of life in line with everyone's wishes, even in the most complex situations.

Chapter 13:
THE PREVENTIVE AND EDUCATIONAL ASPECT FOR PATIENTS

Prevention of vascular diseases

Vascular diseases, which encompass a whole range of conditions linked to the blood vessels, are a major public health issue. The prevalence of these diseases tends to increase with age, but factors such as lifestyle also play a major role. Fortunately, thanks to a better understanding of the underlying causes, many preventive strategies can be adopted to minimise the risks.

Vascular disease: a silent threat
Often insidious, vascular diseases can develop without any obvious symptoms for long periods. When they do occur, they can have serious or even fatal consequences, such as strokes, heart attacks or aneurysms.

Main risk factors :
- **Arterial hypertension:** One of the main culprits when it comes to vascular pathologies.
- **Smoking:** The components of tobacco can damage the vascular walls and accelerate the process of atherosclerosis.
- **Diabetes:** Favours vascular lesions, particularly in the lower limbs.
- **Hyperlipidaemia:** High levels of cholesterol can lead to deposition on the walls of the arteries, forming atherosclerotic plaques.
- **Sedentary lifestyle and obesity:** Promoters of all the above-mentioned risk factors.

Preventive strategies: A path to vascular health
- **Adopting a balanced diet:** Favouring foods rich in fibre, low in saturated fats and sugars, and increasing consumption of fruit, vegetables and fish.
- **Regular physical activity:** At least 30 minutes of moderate activity, such as brisk walking, at least 5 times a week.
- **Stop smoking:** Find resources and help to stop smoking.
- **Weight control:** Maintaining a healthy weight reduces the risk of vascular disease.
- **Stress management:** Adopt relaxation techniques such as meditation or yoga.
- **Medical monitoring:** Regular checks are carried out to monitor and regulate blood pressure, blood sugar levels and cholesterol.
- **Medication:** Take the medication prescribed to treat or prevent vascular disease, always under medical supervision.

Awareness-raising and education :

Educating the general public about the dangers of vascular disease and the importance of prevention is crucial. Awareness campaigns, educational workshops and regular screening can play a decisive role in reducing the incidence of these diseases.

Preventing vascular disease requires an active commitment to a healthy lifestyle. By combining a balanced diet, regular physical activity, appropriate medical supervision and avoiding risky behaviour, it is entirely possible to significantly reduce the risk of developing these devastating diseases. A proactive approach not only benefits vascular health, but also improves overall quality of life.

Promoting healthy lifestyles

Each of us has probably heard the adage "a healthy mind in a healthy body". However, with the rapid pace of modern society and the constant demands on our time and energy, maintaining a healthy lifestyle can seem a daunting challenge. Yet promoting a healthy lifestyle is essential to preventing many chronic diseases, particularly vascular disease, and ensuring a better quality of life.

The multidimensionality of health :
Health is not simply the absence of disease. It encompasses physical, mental and social well-being. So promoting a healthy lifestyle means tackling these different aspects holistically.

The pillars of a healthy lifestyle :
- **Balanced diet:** Eat a varied and balanced diet, giving priority to fresh, local and seasonal foods. Reduce your consumption of ultra-processed foods rich in sugar, salt and saturated fats.
- **Physical activity:** Regular physical activity adapted to your abilities and preferences. This can range from a daily walk to more intense activities such as running or cycling.
- **Quality sleep:** Ensuring a good night's sleep is essential. Insufficient or poor-quality sleep can have harmful consequences for mental and physical health.
- **Stress management:** Learn to identify sources of stress and develop coping mechanisms. This can involve practising meditation or yoga, or simply taking time out.
- **Social interaction:** Positive social relationships are good for mental health. It is important to feel supported and understood.
- **Avoid harmful substances:** Reduce or eliminate consumption of tobacco, alcohol and other drugs.

These substances increase the risk of developing many diseases.

The importance of health education :

It is essential to educate people from an early age about the importance of a healthy lifestyle. Schools, the media, health professionals and public institutions all have a role to play in this education.

Obstacles to healthy living :

Recognising the barriers to adopting a healthy lifestyle is the first step in overcoming them. These may relate to the environment, habits inherited from the family, lack of information or the limited availability of healthy resources.

Promoting healthy lifestyles is more than just a mantra; it's an absolute necessity in our modern world. By putting health at the heart of our concerns and making informed choices, we can not only improve our own well-being, but also that of our community.

Importance of regular monitoring

In the complex journey that is health, regular check-ups are like beacons lighting our way, ensuring that we stay on the right track. Much more than just medical appointments, these key moments map out our health, offering a clear vision of any pitfalls and the best directions to take.

Modern medicine, with its range of advanced technologies, offers remarkably accurate diagnoses. However, it is the regularity of consultations and check-ups that really enables abnormalities to be detected at an early stage, when they are generally easier to treat. This turns regular visits to a doctor or specialist into a proactive line of defence against the development of potentially serious illnesses.

Regular monitoring goes far beyond simply detecting illnesses. They encourage an ongoing dialogue between patient and healthcare professional. This interaction creates a relationship of trust, where the patient feels listened to, understood and cared for. The patient then becomes an active player in his or her own health, involved and aware of the importance of following the recommendations and treatments prescribed.

It is also an opportunity to assess the effectiveness of a treatment in progress, to adjust doses or even to change them if necessary. It's an adaptive approach that adapts to the patient's changing needs, guaranteeing optimal care at every stage of his or her life.

The educational aspect of follow-up care should not be forgotten. They provide an opportunity to inform patients about the latest medical advances, new recommendations and healthier lifestyle habits. The transmission of knowledge is a powerful tool, transforming patients into true guardians of their health.
The importance of regular check-ups cannot be underestimated. They form the solid foundations of a preventive, proactive and adaptive approach to health. In this ballet of consultations and dialogue, each individual, armed with knowledge and supported by his or her healthcare professional, dances gracefully along the path to well-being and longevity.

Chapter 14:
THE INTEGRATION OF TELEMEDICINE

The benefits and effectiveness of telemedicine in vascular surgery

Over the decades, medicine has continued to evolve, shaping and reinventing itself in line with technological advances. Recently, one of the most significant breakthroughs has been telemedicine, enabling care to be delivered remotely using digital tools. In vascular surgery, this innovation has proved remarkably useful and effective, pushing back the traditional boundaries of medical care.

Telemedicine in vascular surgery, as in other disciplines, has proved to be an essential tool, particularly for populations far from specialist care centres. It enables effective post-operative follow-up without the patient having to travel long distances. Images, scans and data can be transmitted in real time, enabling surgeons to assess recovery, detect any complications and adjust treatment recommendations.

In addition to post-operative monitoring, telemedicine is also a valuable tool for **pre-operative consultation**. Patients can benefit from expert advice even if they are geographically distant. This optimises decisions about surgery and prepares the ground for a successful outcome.

One of the major benefits of telemedicine is the **continuing education of** healthcare professionals. Thanks to this technology, surgeons from all over the world can collaborate, sharing complex cases, exchanging innovative surgical techniques and taking part in real-time simulations. Telemedicine acts as a bridge, linking the brilliant minds in vascular surgery and encouraging a collective increase in skills.

However, as promising as it is, telemedicine is not without its challenges. There are questions about **data security**, system interoperability and connection quality, particularly in remote areas. What's more, human contact remains irreplaceable, and some patients may feel a certain distance in this digitised approach.

Telemedicine in vascular surgery has demonstrated its immense potential, opening up new avenues for care, training and collaboration. Although this advance must be approached with caution, it undoubtedly embodies the fusion of technology and medicine, taking vascular surgery to new horizons.

Training and skills required for the nurse

The nursing profession is at the heart of the healthcare system, playing a crucial role in patient care. In vascular surgery, the demands are even more specific, requiring a combination of technical expertise, in-depth medical knowledge and exceptional human qualities.

1. Academic training :
It all starts with **initial training in nursing**. Depending on the country, this may be a nursing diploma, a bachelor's degree or a master's degree. This training includes both theoretical courses and clinical placements, giving students their first exposure to the world of hospitals.

2. Specialisation in vascular surgery :
After gaining general clinical experience, those wishing to specialise in vascular surgery can pursue further training or residencies in this field. They will then learn in detail about

the vascular system, specific surgical procedures, and the pre- and post-operative management of patients.

3. Technical skills :

- **Mastery of specific tools and equipment:** Nurses must be comfortable with a variety of medical instruments, from catheters to cardiac monitors.
- **Preparing the patient for surgery:** This includes placing venous access ports, preparing the skin and monitoring vital signs.
- **Assistance during operations:** Although the surgeon conducts the procedure, the nurse plays a key role in assisting, providing the necessary instruments and monitoring the patient.

4. Clinical skills :

Nurses must be able to rapidly assess a patient's condition, recognise the warning signs of complications and make informed decisions in an emergency situation.

5. Interpersonal skills :

- **Communication:** Nurses are often the first point of contact for patients. They must therefore be able to explain procedures, answer questions and reassure patients and their families.
- **Empathy and compassion:** The ability to put yourself in the patient's shoes, to understand their fears and concerns, is essential.

6. Teamwork :

Vascular surgery is a team effort. Nurses must therefore be able to work effectively with surgeons, anaesthetists, technicians and all medical staff.

7. Commitment to continuing education :

Medicine is a constantly evolving field. Nurses must therefore be prepared to update their skills regularly, take new training courses and adapt to technological and methodological innovations.

The vascular surgery nurse is much more than a simple operator. They are a pillar of the care process, combining technical know-how, clinical expertise and human qualities to ensure the best possible patient care.

Challenges and benefits of this approach

Specialising in vascular surgery offers many opportunities, but it also comes with its share of challenges. Every day, these professionals are faced with a range of complex clinical situations while being at the forefront of technological and medical developments.

Challenges :
- **Increasing complexity of cases:** With advances in medicine, patients who are taken into care may have multiple co-morbidities, making their management more delicate.
- **Continuous updating:** Vascular surgery is a constantly evolving field, requiring nurses to be at the cutting edge of new techniques, drugs and best practice.
- **Emotional burden:** Faced with situations that are often critical, managing your emotions while offering support to patients and their families can be trying.
- **Irregular working hours:** The urgent nature of some vascular interventions means that nurses can often work unexpected hours, including nights and weekends.
- **Pressure and stress:** The need to act quickly, sometimes in life-and-death situations, can generate high levels of stress.

Advantages :
- **Professional satisfaction:** Nothing is more gratifying than seeing a patient recover after successful surgery, knowing that you played a crucial role in that success.

- **Professional development opportunities:** The specialisation offers numerous opportunities for continuing education, participation in research or collaboration with world-renowned experts.
- **Competitive remuneration: Due to** the specialised nature of their role, vascular surgery nurses are often better paid than their counterparts in other fields.
- **Interdisciplinarity:** Working closely with surgeons, anaesthetists, radiologists and other specialists offers an enriching perspective and a holistic approach to care.
- **Direct impact on patients' quality of life:** By helping to restore circulation or avoiding serious vascular complications, nurses have a tangible impact on patients' quality of life.

Although the road to specialising in vascular surgery is littered with challenges, it offers in return invaluable rewards, both professionally and personally. The key lies in continuing education, peer support and an unwavering passion for the well-being of patients.

Chapter 15:
SPECIAL CASES AND SPECIFIC POPULATIONS

Paediatric vascular surgery: specific features and challenges

Paediatric vascular surgery is distinguished by its focus on a very specific demographic group: children, from newborns to adolescents. These patients present unique anatomical, physiological and emotional challenges. Let's take a look at the specific features and challenges of this sub-specialty of vascular surgery.

Special features:
- **Changing anatomy and physiology:** Children's anatomy is constantly changing. The vessels of a newborn or infant are significantly smaller than those of an adolescent or adult. In addition, physiological responses, such as coagulation, differ between children and adults.
- **Unique pathologies:** Certain vascular disorders are specific to the paediatric population, such as certain congenital malformations.
- **Emotional and psychological aspects:** Children may find it difficult to understand what is happening to them, which can lead to anxiety or fear. Parents also play a key role in the decision-making and care process.
- **Medicines and dosages:** Medicines, their dosages and side effects should be adjusted according to the child's weight and age.

Challenges :
- **Communication:** Explaining a procedure or treatment to a child requires an approach that is

adapted to the child's age, maturity and understanding.
- **Comprehensive care:** The approach must be holistic, taking into account not only the medical aspects but also the child's emotional, social and educational needs.
- **Coordination with other specialities:** Children with vascular disorders may also present with other pathologies, requiring close collaboration with other paediatric specialists.
- **Technological developments:** Surgical equipment and instruments must be adapted to the size and fragility of children, which requires specific technological advances.
- **Training and skills: It is** crucial that paediatric vascular surgeons receive specific training to understand and meet the needs of this population.
- **Emotional support:** Providing support for parents, who are often anxious or upset, is just as essential as caring for their child.

Paediatric vascular surgery, while a rewarding speciality, presents its own challenges that require special delicacy, patience and expertise. Every operation, every consultation is an opportunity to transform a life in the making, to give a child the chance to grow up healthy and to reach his or her full potential.

Care for the elderly

Care for the elderly is complex and multidimensional, reflecting the physiological, psychological and social changes that occur with age. The aim is not simply to treat illnesses or symptoms, but to promote optimum quality of life through personalised care that respects the dignity of the individual.

Physiological aspects :
- **Changes to the body:** With age comes changes to the muscles, bones, skin and organ systems, requiring specific, tailored care.
- **Polypathology:** Elderly people often have several illnesses at the same time, requiring a comprehensive approach and coordinated care.
- **Pharmacology:** Drug metabolism changes with age, which can influence dosage and the risk of drug interactions.

Psychological aspects :
- **Memory and cognition:** disorders such as dementia or Alzheimer's disease require special care approaches.
- **Emotional well-being:** Depression, anxiety and loneliness can affect the elderly, which is why psychological and social care is so important.
- **Self-esteem:** Ageing can lead to a decline in self-esteem, linked to physical changes, loss of autonomy or dependence.

Social aspects :
- **Isolation:** Many senior citizens live alone, far from their families or have lost close relatives, increasing the risk of isolation.
- **Autonomy and independence:** Encouraging autonomy and independence, however limited, is essential for the well-being of the elderly.
- **Environment:** Adapted, safe and accessible housing is crucial to preventing falls and promoting independence.

Specialist care :
- **Rehabilitation:** After illness or surgery, appropriate rehabilitation is essential if you are to regain maximum independence.
- **Palliative care:** When a cure is not possible, the focus is on quality of life, comfort and emotional support.

- **Home care:** For those who want it and whose condition allows it, home care is a valuable alternative to hospitalisation or admission to a retirement home.

The key to caring for the elderly lies in a holistic approach that takes account of all the individual's needs. This involves close collaboration between health professionals, social workers, families and communities to ensure comprehensive, respectful and dignified care.

Adapting care for at-risk populations

Navigating the medical field as a nurse involves a heightened sensitivity to the nuances of the diverse populations with whom we interact. More than ever, it is imperative to understand how to adapt care to at-risk populations, thereby ensuring equity and justice in health for all.

Identifying populations at risk :
- **Definition:** These are groups who have a greater likelihood of developing diseases or conditions due to a combination of biological, socio-economic, psychological and environmental factors.
- **Typical examples:** people on low incomes, ethnic minorities, refugees, disabled people, LGBT+ people, people living in remote rural areas, etc.

Understanding the specific challenges :
- **Access to care:** Economic, cultural or geographical barriers may prevent these groups from accessing the care they need.
- **Stigma:** Some groups may be reluctant to seek care because of stigma or discrimination.

- **Language barriers:** Non-native populations may have difficulty understanding medical information or communicating with healthcare staff.
- **Socio-economic factors:** Living conditions, employment, education and socio-economic status can influence a person's health and ability to undergo treatment.

Strategies for adapting care :
- **Cultural training:** Making medical staff aware of different cultures and beliefs to avoid misunderstandings and provide respectful care.
- **Effective communication:** using interpreters, visual aids and adapted teaching aids to overcome language barriers.
- **Working with community organisations:** Working in tandem with community groups can help build trust and improve access to care.
- **Patient-centred approach:** This means considering each patient as a unique individual, recognising and respecting their beliefs, values, life context and preferences.

Continuous assessment and improvement :
- **Patient feedback:** Gather regular feedback from at-risk populations to better understand their needs and adjust care accordingly.
- **Monitoring disparities:** Analysing data to identify disparities in health outcomes and develop targeted interventions.
- **Ongoing training:** Regular training for healthcare staff on best practice in adapted care.

Adapting care to at-risk populations is not only a question of ethics, but also of medical efficiency. By treating each individual with respect, empathy and understanding, we can ensure that every patient receives the best possible care.

Chapter 16:
EMERGENCY VASCULAR SURGERY

Recognising a vascular emergency

In the complex world of medicine, the vascular system - our arteries, veins and capillaries - plays a vital role. Just as a motorway carries vital goods across a country, our blood vessels transport blood, oxygen and nutrients to every nook and cranny of our bodies. When these bloodways experience a problem, it can quickly become a medical emergency. Recognising these vascular emergencies is essential to ensuring timely care and potentially saving a life.

Key symptoms of vascular emergencies :
- **Pain:** Sudden, intense pain may indicate occlusion or trauma to a blood vessel.
- **Pallor or cyanosis:** A limb that becomes pale, bluish or cold may indicate a lack of blood circulation.
- **Weakness or paralysis:** If a major artery in the brain is blocked, this can lead to stroke symptoms.
- **Swelling:** Sudden swelling of a limb can be a sign of deep vein thrombosis.
- **Absence of pulse:** Not feeling the pulse in an area where it would normally be perceptible is a sign of emergency.
- **Signs of bleeding:** External bleeding or signs of internal bleeding such as abdominal pain, distension or fainting.

Common types of vascular emergencies :
- **Dissecting aortic aneurysm:** A tear in the wall of the body's largest artery, which can cause intense pain and requires immediate intervention.

- **Deep vein thrombosis:** The formation of a blood clot in a deep vein, often in the leg.
- **Pulmonary embolism:** When a blood clot travels to the lungs, blocking circulation.
- **Acute limb ischaemia:** A sudden reduction in blood flow to a limb, which may threaten the viability of that limb.

Rapid intervention is the key:
When a vascular emergency is suspected, time is of the essence. Rapid intervention can prevent permanent damage to tissues and organs and even save a patient's life. For healthcare professionals, this means knowing when to refer a patient quickly to vascular surgery specialists or to an emergency department.

The ability to recognise a vascular emergency quickly is based on a combination of theoretical knowledge, clinical observation and medical intuition. Every second counts, and attention to detail can make all the difference to a patient's outcome.

Protocols and rapid intervention

In the world of medicine, where every second can count, knowing how to react quickly and effectively to an emergency situation is crucial. In vascular surgery, this emergency often takes the form of acute circulatory distress, whether due to occlusion, haemorrhage or some other abnormality. It is therefore essential that healthcare professionals, particularly nurses, understand the protocols and procedures to be implemented.

Identifying the emergency :
The first step towards a successful intervention is to quickly recognise the nature of the emergency. This

involves an accurate assessment of the patient, taking into account vital signs, tissue appearance, the presence or absence of a pulse in the affected areas, and any relevant symptoms.

Mobilising the team :
As soon as an emergency is identified, the medical team must be mobilised. This may include the vascular surgeon, anaesthetist, nurses and any other necessary personnel. Clear and effective communication is key at this stage to ensure that everyone is on the same wavelength.

Setting up the emergency protocol :
Each medical institution will have specific protocols for dealing with vascular emergencies. These protocols have generally been developed in line with current best medical practice and are designed to offer the patient the best chance of recovery.

Common rapid vascular surgery procedures include:
- **Restoration of perfusion:** For acute arterial occlusions, this could mean the use of thrombolytic drugs, or mechanical interventions to eliminate a clot.
- **Controlling haemorrhage: In the event** of active bleeding, techniques such as the use of haemostatic dressings, suturing or even the use of forceps may be necessary.
- **Stabilisation and support: Once** the immediate emergency has been managed, the patient may require support in the form of blood transfusions, medication to support blood pressure, or other interventions.

Training and preparation :
The key to success in managing vascular emergencies is preparation. Nurses and other healthcare professionals must be regularly trained in the latest techniques and protocols. Emergency simulations can also be invaluable, allowing teams to practise responding to stressful situations in a controlled environment.

Rapid protocols and interventions in vascular surgery are designed to save lives. Whether it's restoring circulation to a limb or stopping a massive haemorrhage, speed, efficiency and skill are essential to ensure the best outcome for the patient.

Managing post-emergency recovery

After emergency vascular surgery, the recovery period is just as crucial. It requires careful monitoring, meticulous management and clear communication with the patient and his family. The post-emergency phase is a time when nurses play a key role, providing not only physiological care but also psychological support.

Constant clinical monitoring :
Immediately after the operation, the patient is likely to be in a vulnerable state. Regular assessment of vital signs, monitoring of blood oxygenation, and early detection of potential complications such as haemorrhage or infection are essential.

Pain management :
Post-operative pain can be a major concern. Nurses must regularly assess the patient's level of pain, administer analgesics as prescribed and be vigilant about the side effects of these drugs.

Wound care :
Post-operative care involves regular cleansing, assessment of the wound for signs of infection and, possibly, dressing changes. It is crucial to inform the patient of the importance of this care to minimise the risk of infection.

Rehabilitation and physiotherapy :
Depending on the nature of the operation, the patient may require rehabilitation to regain optimal mobility or to strengthen the affected areas. Collaboration with physiotherapists can prove invaluable in this respect.

Psychological support :
A surgical emergency can be a traumatic event for the patient. Listening, patience and the ability to reassure are essential to help the patient navigate through this experience. In some cases, referral to a mental health professional may be beneficial.

Education and follow-up :
Before discharge, the nurse must ensure that the patient and his or her family fully understand the postoperative instructions. This may include medication to be taken, activities to be avoided, signs of complications to be monitored, and the planning of follow-up visits.

Communication with the medical team :
Liaison with surgeons, anaesthetists and other members of the medical team is essential. Any changes in the patient's condition or any concerns must be communicated promptly.

The post-emergency recovery phase is a period when the role of the nurse transcends the simple clinical aspect. It is a mixture of medical expertise, compassion, education and collaboration. By managing this period effectively, the nurse can not only help the patient to heal physically, but also regain confidence in themselves and their future.

Chapter 17:
PALLIATIVE CARE IN VASCULAR SURGERY

When surgery is no longer an option

Sometimes, despite technological advances and the skills of the surgeon, surgery is not an option for a patient. At such times, delicate medical and emotional care is required, and nurses play a central role in accompanying patients and their families through this difficult period.

Understanding the situation:
There may be several reasons why surgery is no longer an option: the risks are too high, the patient's state of health is fragile, the disease is progressing, or the patient himself refuses. In all cases, understanding the medical and emotional reasons behind the decision is essential.

Alternative treatments:
Even without surgery, other treatments may be considered: medication, non-invasive therapies, palliative care. These alternatives can help to manage symptoms, improve quality of life or slow the progression of the disease.

Emotional support:
The news that surgery is no longer an option can come as a shock to patients and their families. Nurses have a duty to provide psychological support, to listen to their worries and fears, and to help them deal with the complex emotions that may arise.

Decision-making:
The patient, in consultation with their family and the medical team, will need to make decisions about the next steps. This could include continuing other treatments, accepting palliative care, or even preparing for the end of life.

Palliative care:
When a cure is no longer an option, the focus shifts to the patient's comfort and quality of life. Palliative care aims to manage pain and symptoms and offer emotional and spiritual support.

Communication with the family:
The family plays a central role in supporting the patient. The nurse must facilitate communication between the patient, the family and the medical team, ensuring that all parties are informed and involved in the decision-making process.

Preparing for the end of life:
If the patient is terminally ill, the nurse can help prepare the patient and their family for this eventuality. This includes discussions about the patient's wishes, the organisation of end-of-life care, and emotional support during this period.

The period when surgery is no longer an option is undoubtedly one of the most trying in a patient's care. It requires multi-dimensional management, with clinical care, emotional support and communication playing equally vital roles. In this ordeal, the nurse often emerges as the central pillar, providing comfort, guidance and expertise at every stage.

Psychological support and symptom relief

Despite its highly technical and specialised nature, vascular surgery is not just about scalpels and sutures. At the heart of this discipline lies the patient and his or her feelings. As a result, both emotional and clinical support are essential to ensure optimal recovery.

The human being behind the patient:
Before being a patient, a patient is an individual with fears,

worries and hopes. The anticipation of surgery, or post-operative recovery, can be a source of stress and anxiety. The nurse is often the first point of contact, the one who takes the hand and reassures.

Listening for better care :
Active listening is one of nurses' most valuable skills. By listening to the patient's concerns, symptoms and even what has not been said, nurses are able to provide appropriate responses, whether medical, informative or simply comforting.

Pain management strategies :
Pain is one of the most commonly encountered symptoms. It can be managed by regular assessment, appropriate medication and non-medicinal techniques such as relaxation, distraction and meditation.

The power of words:
Sometimes talking, putting words to one's ailments, helps us to understand them better. An informed patient who understands his illness and the surgical process is often more serene. Nurses play the role of educator, of translator between medical jargon and everyday language.

Collaboration with mental health professionals:
Some patients may require more in-depth psychological care, beyond the nurse's remit. In these cases, close collaboration with psychologists or psychiatrists is essential.

Holistic care:
Beyond the body, the whole being is taken into account. Spirituality, beliefs, culture - these are all dimensions that can influence the perception of illness and care. As part of their holistic approach, nurses take these various aspects into account to provide tailored, personalised care.

Vascular surgery, like many other medical disciplines, is not limited to a physical operation. Psychological support and the alleviation of symptoms are key elements in the management of the patient, enabling them to live through this ordeal in the best possible conditions. In this delicate ballet between body and mind, the nurse is the intermediary, the guide, the one who ensures the smooth transition between the medical world and the patient's experience.

Collaboration with palliative care teams

Despite its resolute focus on intervention and repair, vascular surgery, like all specialities, comes up against the limits of medicine. When surgery is no longer an option, or when the patient's disease is progressing unfavourably, the approach changes. It becomes less interventionist and more focused on the patient's comfort and quality of life. It is in this context that collaboration with palliative care teams becomes essential.

The importance of communication:
The interface between the vascular surgery team and palliative care requires fluid communication. Each professional brings his or her own expertise to the table, and it is essential that everyone is on the same page when it comes to the care plan and therapeutic objectives.

From intervention to support :
The role of the vascular surgery nurse is changing. Whereas in the past the emphasis was on preparation for surgery and post-operative recovery, it is now shifting towards symptom relief, pain management and, above all, emotional and psychological support for the patient and his or her family.

Humanising the end of life:
Palliative care teams are experts in the art of humanising the end of life. They bring a patient-centred approach, integrating the patient's wishes, fears and beliefs. This

vision is crucial to providing a dignified and serene end of life, even in a hospital environment.

Continuing education and skills exchange:
Collaboration is not only beneficial for the patient. It also offers professionals an opportunity to exchange ideas, learn from each other and enhance their skills. Vascular surgery nurses can learn about palliative care techniques, and conversely, the palliative care team can gain a better understanding of the issues and specifics of vascular surgery.

Respect for choice and autonomy :
The patient, at the heart of this approach, retains his or her autonomy and right to make informed choices. Whether refusing an operation, opting for a less aggressive approach or choosing where to spend their final moments, every decision is respected and honoured.

The collaboration between vascular surgery nurses and palliative care teams is a perfect illustration of the complementary nature of medicine. Each speciality, with its technical skills, expertise and humanity, works together to offer patients a harmonious, respectful and caring care pathway. In this delicate dance between life and the end of life, the nurse is the essential link, the person who ensures that each stage is carried out with dignity and compassion.

Chapter 18:
HEALTHCARE-ASSOCIATED INFECTIONS

Infection prevention

Vascular surgery, with its delicate and often invasive procedures, is particularly sensitive to the issue of infections. Infections can have serious consequences for the patient, prolonging convalescence and sometimes even compromising the success of the operation. Vascular surgery nurses are the first line of defence against the threat of infection, thanks to their rigorous practices and constant vigilance.

Understanding the risk :
One of the first steps in infection prevention is to fully understand the associated risks. Vascular surgery patients may have underlying conditions, such as diabetes, that make them more vulnerable. In addition, the use of vascular implants or prostheses can also increase the risk of infection.

Hand hygiene: the essential gesture :
The simplicity of this gesture should not mask its crucial importance. Thorough and regular hand washing, before and after each contact with the patient, is one of the most effective measures for preventing the transmission of infectious agents.

Proper use of personal protective equipment (PPE):
Gloves, gowns, masks and goggles are only effective if they are used correctly. It is therefore vital for nurses to be familiar with the protocols for their use and to ensure that they are scrupulously observed.

Monitoring entry points:
Incision sites, catheters, or any other point of entry into the body can be entry points for bacteria. Nurses should

regularly monitor these areas, looking for signs of infection such as redness, heat, pain or discharge.

Patient training and education :
The patient is a key player in infection prevention. Nurses must therefore ensure that patients and their families are aware of the signs of infection, the hygiene measures to be followed, and the importance of reporting any suspicious symptoms promptly.

Disinfection protocols :
Equipment, instruments and surfaces in the hospital environment must be regularly disinfected according to strict protocols to minimise the risk of contamination.

Preventing infections in vascular surgery is a constant battle, requiring rigour, training and vigilance. Nurses, by virtue of their central role in patient care and their proximity to the patient, are key players in this preventive approach. Through their interventions and vigilance, they actively contribute to ensuring patient safety and the success of surgical procedures.

Management and processing post-operative infections

In vascular surgery, a post-operative infection is more than just an inconvenience. It represents a potential threat to the success of the operation, to the patient's well-being, and can sometimes have fatal consequences. Rapid management, accurate diagnosis and appropriate treatment are therefore essential.

Early recognition of signs :
Post-operative infection often manifests itself through classic symptoms: redness, heat, pain and swelling at the surgical site, but also fever, chills or a purulent discharge.

Nurses must be trained to recognise these signs quickly and to act without delay.

Sampling and diagnosis:
At the slightest suspicion of infection, samples are taken to identify the pathogen responsible. This enables antibiotic treatment to be targeted. Medical imaging can also be used to assess the extent of the infection.

Rapid medical intervention:
Medical treatment must be immediate. It often begins with the administration of broad-spectrum antibiotics, pending the results of swabs. If a collection of pus is present, surgery may be required to drain the abscess.

Specific nursing care :
As well as administering the prescribed treatments, nurses play a crucial role in monitoring the progress of the infection. They must ensure rigorous asepsis of wounds, keep the surgical site clean and disinfected, and regularly monitor the patient's vital parameters.

Patient education and advice:
Patients and their families must be informed of the importance of monitoring the surgical site for signs of infection. They should also be trained to carry out local care, if necessary, and made aware of the importance of scrupulously following the antibiotic treatment prescribed.

Preventing recurrence:
Once a post-operative infection has been treated, regular monitoring is essential to prevent recurrences. This involves check-ups, blood tests and, if necessary, adjustments to treatment.

Managing post-operative infections in vascular surgery is a major challenge for patient safety. Thanks to their expertise, vigilance and proximity to patients, nurses are at the forefront of this battle. Their role in recognising, treating and preventing infections is therefore absolutely central.

The challenges of resistance antibiotics

The discovery of antibiotics in the 20th century revolutionised modern medicine, offering a powerful remedy for a host of previously often fatal infections. Over time, however, an unforeseen threat developed: antibiotic resistance. This phenomenon grew rapidly and became a major issue for all areas of medicine, including vascular surgery.

1. Understanding antibiotic resistance :
Antibiotic resistance occurs when bacteria develop the ability to overcome the effects of drugs designed to kill or inhibit them. This may be the result of natural mutation or adaptation to repeated exposure to antibiotics. These resistant bacteria multiply and spread, making infections more difficult to treat.

2. Implications for vascular surgery :
Vascular surgery, which treats disorders of the blood vessels, is not immune to infection. Whether these are post-operative infections or infections linked to medical devices such as catheters, antibiotic resistance complicates treatment, prolongs recovery time, increases the cost of care and raises the risk of morbidity and mortality.

3. Current practice and risks :
Prophylactic antibiotics are commonly used in vascular surgery to prevent infections. However, their inappropriate or excessive use can contribute to resistance. In addition, prescribing antibiotics post-operatively, without a clear rationale, can exacerbate the problem.

4. The need for stewardship :
Antibiotic stewardship is essential to combat resistance. It aims to ensure that antibiotics are used judiciously, only when necessary and with the right agent, dose, route and duration.

5. Interdisciplinary collaboration :
Combating antibiotic resistance requires a collaborative approach involving surgeons, infectiologists, pharmacologists and nurses. Together, they can develop and implement protocols to ensure the appropriate use of antibiotics.

6. Educate and raise awareness:
It is vital to educate medical staff, patients and the public about the dangers of antibiotic resistance and the importance of using these medicines responsibly.

Antibiotic resistance is one of the most pressing challenges facing modern medicine. In vascular surgery, where the risk of infection is omnipresent, the need to address this problem is even more acute. It is imperative to combine research, education and collaboration to safeguard the efficacy of these vital medicines for future generations.

Chapter 19:
RAPID RECOVERY AFTER SURGERY (RRAC)

Principles of the RRAC in vascular surgery

Rapid Enhanced Recovery After Surgery (RRAS) is a multidisciplinary approach to improving patients' recovery from surgery. It is based on a series of predefined protocols that seek to minimise surgical stress and promote a rapid return to normal function. Although RRAC was initially developed for colorectal surgery, its principles have been adapted to other surgical fields, including vascular surgery. Here are the main aspects of RRAC applied to vascular surgery:

1. Preoperative assessment and preparation:
   - **Nutritional assessment:** Identifying and treating malnutrition to improve post-operative outcomes.
   - **Medical optimisation:** Management of co-morbidities such as diabetes, hypertension and heart disease.
   - **Patient education:** Inform the patient about the surgical process, recovery expectations and the importance of early mobilisation.
   - **Prehabilitation:** physical, nutritional and psychological reinforcement of the patient before the operation.
2. Anaesthesia and analgesia:
   - **Locoregional anaesthesia:** Favoured whenever possible to reduce the side effects of general anaesthetics.

- **Multimodal pain management:** Combined use of analgesics to optimise pain relief while reducing opioids.

3. Surgical techniques to minimise trauma:
   - **Minimal surgical access:** Favour endovascular techniques or small incisions where appropriate.
   - **Prevention of blood loss:** Use of techniques and tools to reduce bleeding.

4. Post-operative:
   - **Early mobilisation:** Encourage the patient to get up and move around as soon as possible after the operation.
   - **Early feeding:** Rapid reintroduction of a normal diet.
   - **Limitation of drains and catheters:** rapid removal to encourage mobility and reduce the risk of infection.
   - **Management of nausea and vomiting:** Use of antiemetic drugs to prevent and treat symptoms.

5. Post-operative follow-up :
   - **Discharge criteria:** Define clear criteria for hospital discharge.
   - **Follow-up at home:** Follow-up to identify and quickly manage any complications.

6. Continuous review :
   - **Audit and feedback:** Regular assessment of RRAC protocols to ensure they are effective and to make improvements.

RRAC in vascular surgery offers an opportunity to improve the quality of care and outcomes for patients. Using a multidisciplinary approach, it aims to minimise surgical trauma, promote rapid recovery and reduce the length of hospital stay.

The key role of the nurse in the RRAC pathway

Rapid Enhanced Rehabilitation (RRAC) is an innovative approach to surgical care. It requires a close-knit, multidisciplinary team, in which the nurse plays a pivotal role. From pre-operative to post-operative follow-up, nurses are at the heart of the implementation and success of RRAC.

1. Patient education and preparation :
The nurse is often the first point of contact for the patient. They are responsible for informing the patient about the procedure and what to expect before, during and after surgery. This pre-operative education is essential to reduce the patient's anxiety and give them the tools they need to play an active part in their recovery.

2. Pre-operative assessment :
The nurse plays a key role in risk assessment and pre-operative preparation. This includes checking medical histories, coordinating with other specialists if necessary, and ensuring that all pre-operative protocols are followed.

3. Intraoperative coordination :
Although the surgical act is primarily in the hands of the surgeon, the operating theatre nurse ensures patient safety, prepares and checks the necessary equipment, and works closely with the anaesthetist and surgeon.

4. Post-operative support :
After surgery, the nurse is essential for monitoring the patient, administering analgesics, ensuring early mobilisation, and encouraging feeding. They are also responsible for recognising and managing potential complications, and coordinating with other members of the team to ensure comprehensive care.

5. Post-operation education :
Before returning home, the nurse reiterates post-operative advice, provides information on signs and symptoms to

watch out for, and reassures the patient about the recovery process. They also offer follow-up resources and answer any questions the patient and family may have.

6. Follow-up :
The nurse is often the first person patients contact if they have any concerns after returning home. They assess the patient's well-being, answer their questions and, if necessary, refer them to the right healthcare professional.

7. Continuous improvement:
As an active member of the surgical team, the nurse also participates in the revision of RRAC protocols, providing valuable feedback for the continuous improvement of care.

In the RRAC pathway, the nurse is much more than just an operator. They are a central pillar of the patient's care, ensuring that every stage of the process is optimised for rapid and effective recovery. Their expertise, compassion and commitment to the patient are essential to the success of the RRAC.

Benefits and challenges of this approach

Rapid Surgical Enhanced Rehabilitation (RRAC) is a multidisciplinary approach that aims to optimise a patient's recovery from surgery, minimising complications and reducing the length of hospital stay. While there are many benefits to implementing RRAC, there are also challenges. Let's take a look at the benefits and obstacles of this approach.

Benefits :
1. Accelerated recovery: RRAC protocols promote faster recovery, enabling patients to regain their independence and quality of life more quickly.
2. Reducing complications: Thanks to better pre-operative preparation and optimised management during

and after surgery, RRAC helps to reduce the risk of post-operative complications.

3. Shorter hospital stays: A rapid recovery also means a shorter hospital stay, which reduces costs and frees up beds for other patients.

4. Patient satisfaction: Better pain management, early mobilisation and clear information improve patient experience and satisfaction.

5. Financial savings: Reducing length of stay and complications can result in significant savings for healthcare establishments.

Challenges :

1. Resistance to change : Implementing a RRAC programme may meet with resistance from healthcare teams used to long-established protocols.

2. Training and education: The success of RRAC requires healthcare professionals to be adequately trained in this approach and to receive ongoing education to keep abreast of developments in the protocols.

3. Multidisciplinary coordination: RRAC requires close collaboration between different healthcare professionals (surgeons, anaesthetists, nurses, physiotherapists, etc.). This coordination can be difficult to establish and maintain.

4. Managing expectations: Properly informing patients about RRAC is crucial to managing their expectations. Some may expect an immediate recovery and be disappointed if this is not the case.

5. Adaptability: Not all patients are eligible for RRAC. It is therefore essential to assess each case individually and adapt the protocol accordingly.

RRAC offers a promising approach to improving surgical outcomes and patient satisfaction. However, its implementation requires careful planning, appropriate training, and interprofessional collaboration to overcome the challenges inherent in this paradigm shift in surgical care.

Chapter 20:
THE FUTURE OF VASCULAR SURGERY: INNOVATIONS AND CHALLENGES

New techniques and materials

Vascular surgery, like other medical fields, is making constant advances thanks to research and innovation. New techniques and materials are emerging to make operations safer, reduce patient recovery times and improve long-term results. Let's take a look at some of the major advances in this field.

1. Endovascular techniques :
These minimally invasive techniques use catheters and other devices inserted through a small incision to treat vascular problems without the need for open surgery. They offer shorter recovery times and fewer post-operative complications.

2. Drug-releasing stents :
Stents, which are tubular devices placed to keep a blood vessel open, are now impregnated with drugs that help prevent restenosis, or narrowing of the vessel after surgery.

3. Biodegradable materials :
These materials offer the advantage of temporarily supporting a vessel while being gradually absorbed by the body. They reduce the risk of long-term complications associated with permanent devices.

4. Real-time 3D imaging :
This technology enables surgeons to accurately visualise the patient's vascular anatomy during the operation, improving the accuracy and safety of the procedure.

5. Surgical robotics :
Increasingly sophisticated robots are assisting surgeons, enabling them to carry out operations with greater precision and even smaller incisions.

6. Biomimicry :
Innovative materials are designed to mimic the structure and function of human tissue, allowing better integration and reducing the risk of rejection or complications.

7. Post-operative monitoring techniques :
New devices allow continuous monitoring of blood flow and vascular health after the operation, guaranteeing rapid intervention in the event of any anomaly.

8. Gene and cell therapies :
Research is continuing into gene and cell therapies to promote vascular repair and regeneration, offering a new way of treating vascular disorders without surgery.

The combination of technology, innovation and medical research continues to propel vascular surgery towards new horizons. These advances, which focus on patient well-being and safety, reinforce the importance of ongoing training for healthcare professionals to ensure they adopt and master these new techniques and materials.

Vascular surgery in the digital age

The advent of the digital age has transformed many disciplines, and vascular surgery is no exception. As digital technologies continue to advance at breakneck speed, their integration into the medical field promises more efficient, precise and personalised care for patients. Let's delve into this fascinating world where technology and medicine meet.

1. Advanced imaging and diagnostics :
Thanks to digital technology, medical imaging such as angiography and computer tomography has reached unprecedented levels of precision. High-resolution images provide vascular surgeons with detailed views of blood vessels, enabling more accurate diagnosis and targeted surgery.

2. Simulation and training :
Digital simulators give surgeons in training the opportunity to perform complex operations in a virtual environment. This enhances their skills, reduces errors and improves patient safety.

3. Robotics and surgical assistance :
Computer-assisted robots are now widely used in vascular surgery. They allow more precise and stable movements than the human hand, while offering better visualisation of the operating area.

4. Electronic medical records :
These systems centralise patient medical information, making it easier for specialists to share information, improving care coordination and reducing medical errors.

5. Telemedicine :
Remote consultation has become a reality. It gives patients access to specialists, even if they live in remote areas. In the vascular field, this can mean remote post-operative monitoring or consultations for second opinions.

6. Applications and wearables :
Wearable devices and mobile applications can now be used to continuously monitor certain vital data, providing a real-time view of a patient's vascular health and alerting them to any abnormalities.

7. Artificial intelligence and data analysis :
AI can help to rapidly analyse large quantities of data, identify trends or anomalies and even suggest treatments. It could revolutionise the early treatment of vascular diseases.

8. 3D printers :
Although still in the experimental phase, 3D printing has the potential to create tailor-made vascular grafts for patients, based on their unique anatomy.

The digital age, with its technological innovations, is pushing back the boundaries of what is possible in vascular surgery. While this presents challenges, particularly in terms of data security and ethics, it also opens up exciting horizons for improving patient care. As healthcare professionals, it is crucial that we adapt to these developments, continually educate ourselves and adopt these tools to offer the best to our patients.

Ethical issues medical innovations

Every major technological advance raises a series of ethical dilemmas. Despite their undeniable benefits in terms of health and quality of life, medical innovations are not exempt from these questions. Doctors, researchers, legislators and even patients find themselves faced with new challenges that require careful thought.

1. Equity and accessibility :
One of the major concerns is the accessibility of new technologies. Who can benefit from these innovations? How can we ensure that medical advances benefit everyone and do not exacerbate socio-economic inequalities?

2. Privacy and data protection :
With the rise of telemedicine, electronic medical records and connected devices, the collection of sensitive data is intensifying. How can the security and confidentiality of this information be guaranteed?

3. Informed consent :

Do patients really understand the implications and risks of new technologies and treatments? How can we ensure that their consent is truly informed, especially when the innovation is **complex?**

4. Experimentation and testing :
Before an innovation is widely adopted, it must be tested. What are the ethical criteria for conducting clinical trials, especially when the technology is radically new?

5. Modulation and improvement of the human body :
With innovations such as genomics and neuronal implants, where do we draw the line between treatment and 'improvement' of the human body? Is it ethical to go beyond simple healing?

6. Genetic interventions :
The possibility of modifying the human genome, in particular with tools such as CRISPR, opens the door to immense opportunities, but also to profound ethical dilemmas, particularly with regard to transgenerational modifications.

7. Artificial intelligence in medicine :
AI has huge potential for diagnosis and treatment, but who is responsible if it goes wrong? How can we ensure that AI makes decisions fairly and without bias?

8. End of life and innovations :
Medical technologies can sometimes prolong life, but at what cost to quality of life? When is it ethical to use or refuse a life-prolonging technology?

Medical innovation is a formidable driver of progress, but it must be guided by sound ethical reflection. The stakes are immense and require collaboration between healthcare professionals, patients, legislators and ethics experts to ensure that technological advances genuinely serve human well-being.

Chapter 21:
TRANSITION BETWEEN HOSPITAL AND HOME

Planning your outing and patient education

The transition between a hospital stay and going home is a key moment in medical care, and this is where nurses play a crucial role. A well-planned discharge and appropriate patient education are essential to ensure a safe convalescence and to reduce the risk of complications or readmissions to hospital.

1. Initial assessment :
The nurse must first assess the patient's state of health, level of understanding, needs and the resources available at home. This assessment will enable the discharge plan to be personalised.

2. Coordination with the medical team :
In collaboration with the doctor, the nurse establishes the care plan to be followed once the patient has returned home. This may include follow-up appointments, medication adjustments or other recommendations.

3. Teaching self-care :
It is vital to educate patients on how to look after themselves. This includes managing medication, recognising warning signs, wound care, recommended physical activity and other specific instructions.

4. Emotional support :
Returning home after surgery or illness can be a source of anxiety. Nurses must offer emotional support, answer

patients' questions and, if necessary, refer them to mental health professionals or support groups.

5. Planning needs at home :
Some patients may need specific equipment at home, such as a medical bed, a walker or other technical aids. The nurse coordinates this.

6. Support network :
Identifying and involving family, friends or informal carers who can help with the patient's care at home is crucial. Training them in the specific tasks the patient needs ensures continuity of care.

7. Community resources :
The nurse can refer the patient to local resources such as homecare services, rehabilitation programmes or patient associations.

8. Follow-up :
Follow-up after discharge, whether by telephone, telemedicine or home visits, ensures that the patient is doing well and complying with medical instructions.

Discharge planning and patient education are crucial steps in ensuring a smooth transition from hospital to home. By investing time and energy in these stages, the nurse plays a decisive role in the patient's well-being and recovery.

Post-operative monitoring at home

After vascular surgery, the recovery phase does not stop once the patient leaves hospital. Post-operative monitoring at home is essential to ensure complete recovery, prevent complications and guarantee the patient's well-being.

1. Initial post-discharge assessment :
As soon as they return home, patients should be aware of the importance of regular assessment of their condition. This includes checking vital signs, monitoring surgical wounds and observing expected postoperative symptoms.

2. Wound monitoring :
The operated area requires special attention. The nurse teaches the patient how to check the wound for signs of infection, haemorrhage or other abnormalities.

3. Pain management :
Pain is a common symptom after surgery. It is essential that the patient knows how to manage pain using prescribed medication and non-pharmacological methods, while remaining alert to possible side effects.

4. Physical activity :
Depending on the nature of the operation, specific recommendations regarding physical activity will be given. It is crucial to follow these guidelines to promote optimal recovery and prevent possible complications.

5. Nutrition and hydration :
Diet can play a decisive role in recovery. Good hydration and a balanced diet help healing and overall recovery.

6. Warning signs :
The patient should be made aware of warning signs or unusual symptoms which should be reported immediately, such as chest pain, sudden weakness, excessive swelling or skin changes.

7. Medication :
Strict adherence to the medication regime is essential. Patients must be aware of schedules, dosages and possible drug interactions.

8. Follow-up visits :
Post-operative appointments with the surgeon or medical team are often necessary to assess the progress of healing.

9. Emotional support :
Surgery can have a psychological impact. Support from

loved ones, or even a professional, can be beneficial in managing postoperative emotions.

Post-operative monitoring at home is a crucial stage in the recovery process. By working closely with healthcare professionals and following guidelines, patients increase their chances of a successful recovery and improved quality of life after surgery.

Working with home care and rehabilitation

The period following surgery is critical, not only for physical recovery, but also for the patient's emotional and psychological recovery. The link between hospital care and care at home, as well as rehabilitation, is essential to ensure a full and high-quality recovery.

1. The transition from hospital to home:
Discharge from hospital is a key moment. It requires precise coordination between the hospital team, the homecare service and the patient's family to ensure that all the necessary resources are in place.

2. Home assessment :
Home care providers carry out an initial assessment to understand the patient's environment, identify specific needs and put in place a suitable care plan.

3. Rehabilitation: a crucial stage :
Vascular surgery may require a period of rehabilitation to regain mobility, strength and endurance. This stage is facilitated by physiotherapists, occupational therapists and other specialists who work closely with the nurse.

4. Monitoring and adapting the care plan :
Depending on the patient's progress, home care and rehabilitation programmes may need to be adjusted. Fluid

communication between all those involved is essential to adapt to changes.

5. Patient education and empowerment:
The nurse, in collaboration with the home care team, plays a vital role in educating the patient and family about post-operative care, medication, nutrition, exercise and other elements essential to recovery.

6. Psychological and social support :
In addition to physiological needs, patients may experience emotional and social challenges following surgery. Psychological support, through professionals or support groups, as well as social support, can be beneficial.

7. Complication management :
Rapid response to any complications is crucial. The nurse, in collaboration with the homecare team, must be vigilant and prepared to act quickly in the event of a problem.

Close collaboration between hospital services, home care and rehabilitation is fundamental to ensuring optimal recovery after vascular surgery. This alliance provides holistic care for patients, addressing their physical, emotional and social needs, while optimising their return to a normal, active life.

Chapter 22:
VASCULAR TRAUMA AND CARE

Initial assessment of trauma

The immediate management of trauma patients is crucial in determining the severity of injuries, establishing an appropriate treatment plan and improving the chances of recovery. The accuracy and speed of this initial assessment can mean the difference between life and death. Here's how this essential stage in the treatment of trauma victims is organised:

1. Ensuring patient safety and stabilisation :
As soon as a trauma patient arrives, the first step is to ensure their safety and that of the medical team. This involves checking the airway, making sure the patient can breathe and stabilising blood circulation.

2. Rapid collection of information :
It is imperative to quickly obtain a history of the trauma. What is the nature of the trauma? How did it happen? Are there other victims? This information can help the medical team to anticipate certain problems and plan the necessary interventions.

3. Primary physical examination :
A rapid but systematic examination is carried out to identify potentially life-threatening injuries. This includes checking vital functions, assessing neurological status and detecting any haemorrhage.

4. Detailed secondary examination :
Once the patient has been stabilised, a more detailed examination is carried out to identify other less obvious but equally serious injuries. This process includes inspection, palpation, percussion and auscultation.

5. Use of diagnostic imaging :
Tools such as radiography, ultrasound, computed

tomography (CT) and magnetic resonance imaging (MRI) can be used to obtain a detailed view of internal injuries.

6. Identification of treatment priorities :
Based on the injuries identified, the medical team prioritises treatment. Some interventions may be required immediately, while others may have to wait.

7. Communication with the patient and family :
It is essential to communicate the results of the assessment to the patient and family, as well as providing information about the next steps in treatment.

Initial trauma assessment is a crucial stage that requires a structured, methodical and rapid approach. The ability to quickly and accurately assess the severity of a trauma can significantly improve a patient's chances of survival and recovery. Collaboration between all members of the medical team is vital to ensure effective and efficient trauma management.

Emergency response and stabilisation

When a crisis arises in vascular surgery, every second counts. Vascular complications can quickly lead to irreversible damage to tissues and organs, or be life-threatening. In these moments of high tension, emergency interventions must be implemented effectively to stabilise the patient and prevent further damage.

1. Rapid assessment :
Before any intervention, a rapid assessment of the patient's condition is essential. This assessment must determine the seriousness of the situation, the organ systems involved, and identify the immediate priorities.

2. Life support :
Emergency interventions often focus on maintaining vital functions. This involves stabilising the airway, ensuring

adequate ventilation, and circulatory resuscitation to ensure adequate organ perfusion.

3. Bleeding control :
In the context of vascular surgery, unexpected bleeding is one of the most common emergencies. Rapid access to the site of bleeding, direct compression, the use of haemostatic devices and, if necessary, surgical intervention may be essential.

4. Administration of emergency drugs :
Depending on the nature of the emergency, drugs such as vasoactive agents, analgesics, or anti-arrhythmic drugs may be administered to stabilise the patient.

5. Surgical intervention :
If non-surgical measures are not sufficient, surgery may be required to resolve the problem. This may include repair of a damaged vessel, removal of a clot, or placement of a shunt.

6. Continuous monitoring :
Once the emergency situation has been managed, constant monitoring of the patient is necessary. Vital parameters, diuresis, oxygenation levels and other vital signs are closely monitored to ensure that the patient remains stable.

7. Psychological support :
The psychological impact of a medical emergency on the patient and those close to them should not be overlooked. Ensuring clear communication and offering psychological support can help reduce anxiety and fear.

Emergency vascular surgery requires a skilled medical team, state-of-the-art equipment and established procedures to manage complications effectively. The main objective is to stabilise the patient as quickly as possible, while minimising the risk of further damage. In these critical moments, coordination, speed of action and expertise are essential to saving lives.

Recovery and rehabilitation post-traumatic

The period following a trauma, particularly in the field of vascular surgery, is crucial. Appropriate care, focusing on recovery and rehabilitation, is essential to ensure that patients make the best possible recovery and gradually return to a normal life.

1. Acute phase: stabilisation and monitoring
Following trauma or emergency vascular surgery, patients are generally admitted to intensive care or a post-operative monitoring unit. The aim of this phase is to stabilise the patient's condition, manage pain, monitor any complications and begin initial rehabilitation care.

2. Multidisciplinary assessment:
A team comprising vascular surgeons, physiotherapists, nutritionists, psychologists and other specialists assesses the patient's specific needs to define an individualised rehabilitation plan.

3. Early mobilisation:
Depending on the nature of the trauma, encouraging early mobilisation can prevent complications, such as thrombosis, and promote faster recovery.

4. Wound care :
Appropriate management of incisions or traumatic wounds is essential to prevent infection, promote optimal healing and minimise scarring.

5. Physical rehabilitation:
Targeted exercises, supervised by a physiotherapist, help to restore strength, mobility and endurance. This is particularly relevant if the trauma has affected the patient's ability to walk or use certain parts of their body.

6. Psychological support :
Trauma can leave emotional scars. Psychological care can help patients deal with shock, fear, anxiety and post-traumatic stress.

7. Patient education:
It is vital to inform patients about their condition, home care, medication and warning signs. This helps them to take control of their own recovery.

8. Long-term follow-up:
Regular appointments with the medical team allow you to monitor the progress of your rehabilitation, adjust your treatments and identify any complications at an early stage.

9. Social and professional reintegration:
Depending on the severity of the trauma, it may take time to return to a normal life. Aids such as occupational therapy, job adjustments or vocational training may be necessary.

Post-trauma recovery and rehabilitation are complex processes that require comprehensive, multidisciplinary care. Medical advances now make it possible to offer increasingly effective treatment aimed at restoring patients' independence and improving their quality of life.

Chapter 23:
DIGITAL TOOLS AND APPLICATIONS FOR NURSES

Tracking software and patient assessment

In the modern medical world, technology plays a key role, particularly in the management and monitoring of patient records. The use of dedicated software offers healthcare professionals an efficient and structured way of monitoring patient progress, assessing their needs and ensuring optimal care.

1. Why is digital monitoring crucial?
Digitalisation has made it possible to centralise information, facilitate access and reduce the risk of error. Paper files are often voluminous and can be lost or incomplete, whereas the right software ensures that patient data can be traced and updated in real time.

2. Characteristics of monitoring software :
- **Intuitive interface:** for fast data entry.
- **Secure access:** Only authorised professionals can access sensitive information.
- **Interoperability:** the software's ability to exchange data with other systems, making it easier to share information between different departments or establishments.
- **Real-time updates:** as soon as new information is added, it is immediately available to the care team.
- **Alert functions:** in the event of an anomaly or the need for urgent intervention.

3. Benefits for the patient :
The software enables personalised, tailored monitoring. Patients benefit from better support and, in some cases,

can have direct access to some of their data, thereby encouraging their involvement in their care.

4. Benefits for nursing staff :
- **Save time:** reduce administrative tasks.
- **Informed decision-making:** rapid access to the patient's complete history.
- **Better coordination:** Facilitates communication between different members of the medical team.

5. Developments and trends :
With the advent of artificial intelligence and telemedicine, medical monitoring software is constantly evolving. They can incorporate predictive analysis functions, diagnostic assistance tools or teleconsultation modules.

6. Ethical and regulatory issues :
The digitisation of medical data raises ethical issues, particularly concerning confidentiality and security. Software publishers and healthcare establishments must comply with strict standards to guarantee data protection.

Patient monitoring and assessment software has become an essential part of the medical landscape. They promote optimal care, tailored to the specific needs of each patient, while facilitating the work of healthcare teams. However, their use requires particular attention to data security and confidentiality.

Use of connected objects in post-operative follow-up

The emergence of connected devices in the medical world has revolutionised patient care, particularly in post-operative monitoring. These devices add a new dimension to the care pathway, making home monitoring more effective and personalised.

1. The era of connected objects in medicine :
Connected objects, or the Internet of Things (IoT) in medicine, refer to medical devices capable of collecting, analysing and transmitting health data in real time, enabling remote monitoring of patients.

2. Types of objects used in post-operative monitoring :
- **Connected watches and bracelets:** measure parameters such as heart rate, body temperature and physical activity.
- **Connected scale:** to monitor the patient's weight, which is particularly important after certain operations.
- **Connected blood pressure monitor:** monitors blood pressure and sends alerts in the event of abnormalities.
- **Patches and skin devices:** can measure a variety of data, from skin hydration to cardiac parameters.

3. Benefits for the patient :
- **Real-time monitoring:** Data is transmitted continuously, enabling rapid intervention in the event of an anomaly.
- **Greater autonomy:** Patients can manage their recovery at home, while remaining connected to their medical team.
- **Motivation:** Visualising progress can be a powerful motivator for patients.

4. Benefits for nursing staff :
- **Access to accurate data:** Connected objects provide regular, reliable measurements.
- **Optimised follow-up:** Remote monitoring reduces the number of post-operative visits, while ensuring high-quality follow-up.
- **Early warnings:** In the event of a complication, the system can quickly detect any warning signs.

5. Challenges and concerns :
- **Data security :** With the proliferation of connected objects, data security and confidentiality must be a priority.
- **Device reliability: It is** crucial that devices provide accurate data to ensure patient safety.
- **Cost:** Although many connected objects are affordable, some can represent a substantial investment.

6. The future of connected devices in vascular surgery:
With the rapid development of technology, we can expect to see the emergence of objects dedicated to specific pathologies or interventions, enabling even more tailored and personalised monitoring.

Connected devices have undeniably transformed the landscape of post-operative monitoring in vascular surgery. They offer exciting opportunities to improve the quality of care and patient satisfaction. However, as with any innovation, they must be used with discernment and in compliance with the rules of confidentiality and medical ethics.

Digital security and data confidentiality

In the age of digital medicine, digital security and data confidentiality have become key issues for the medical sector. Technological advances, while bringing countless benefits, also introduce potential risks that must be managed.

1. Digitalisation in vascular surgery:
The vascular surgery sector, like other medical disciplines, is undergoing a major digital transformation. Electronic medical records, digitised medical imaging, telemedicine

and the use of connected objects are all examples of this transformation.

2. Importance of confidentiality :

The confidentiality of medical data is fundamental. Respecting medical confidentiality is a patient's right, but it is also an obligation for healthcare staff.

3. Risks and threats :

- **Cyber attacks:** Hospitals and clinics can be targeted by attacks aimed at stealing, modifying or rendering inaccessible sensitive information.
- **Human error:** Inadvertent sharing, loss of a device containing data or configuration errors can jeopardise the confidentiality of information.
- **Malicious software:** Some software can infiltrate systems to steal or corrupt data.

4. Protective measures :

- **Staff training:** It is crucial to educate medical and administrative staff about best practice in digital security.
- **Strict protocols:** Implement data access procedures, strong passwords and two-factor verification systems.
- **Regular updates:** Software and systems must be regularly updated to correct vulnerabilities.

5. Legislation and standards :

In many countries, legislation imposes strict standards for the protection of medical data. These laws aim to ensure the confidentiality, integrity and availability of information.

6. Shared responsibility :

The protection of medical data is a shared responsibility between healthcare establishments, technology suppliers and the patients themselves. Each player must be aware of their role and the implications of their actions.

7. The future of digital safety in vascular surgery:

With the advent of technologies such as artificial intelligence and machine learning in medicine, safety challenges are set to become even more complex.

However, with a proactive and collaborative approach, the sector can continue to innovate while protecting patient rights and safety.

As the medical world continues to embrace digital technology, the issue of data security and confidentiality will continue to grow in importance. It is imperative for those involved in vascular surgery, as it is for the medical sector as a whole, to ensure a secure environment for all.

Chapter 24: SPECIALISATIONS AND SUB-DISCIPLINES IN VASCULAR SURGERY

Angiology and venous pathologies

Angiology, often referred to as the science of vessels, is particularly interested in arteries, veins and capillaries. While the arteries have the onerous task of carrying oxygenated blood from the heart to the rest of the body, the veins carry deoxygenated blood back to the heart. However efficient this system may be, it is not immune to malfunction. Let's take a look at the main venous pathologies and the issues involved.

1. What is angiology?
   - Definition and scope of action
   - Interaction with other medical disciplines
   - Diagnostic and therapeutic importance
2. Structure and function of veins :
   - Anatomy of veins: superficial, deep and perforating
   - The role of venous valves
   - The venous return process
3. Common venous pathologies :
   - **Varicose veins:** Permanent dilatation of a vein, often visible on the surface of the skin.
   - **Deep vein thrombosis (DVT):** formation of a blood clot in a deep vein, usually in the legs.
   - **Phlebitis:** Inflammation of a vein, often accompanied by the formation of a blood clot.
   - **Venous insufficiency:** Inability of the veins to ensure an efficient return of blood to the heart.
4. Risk factors and prevention :
   - Heredity, age and gender

- Sedentary lifestyle
- Pregnancy and hormones
- Overweight and obesity
- Preventive advice: physical activity, raising the legs, balanced diet

5. Symptoms and diagnosis :
   - Warning signs: heavy legs, swelling, pain, change in skin colour
   - Clinical examinations: palpation, Doppler ultrasound, phlebography

6. Treatments and interventions :
   - Medication: anticoagulants, anti-inflammatories, venotonics
   - Surgery: stripping, phlebectomy
   - Less invasive techniques: sclerotherapy, endovenous laser, radiofrequency
   - Medical compression: compression stockings and bandages

7. Living with venous disease :
   - Impact on quality of life
   - Day-to-day symptom management
   - Recommendations to avoid complications

Venous pathologies, although common, can have a significant impact on patients' health and quality of life. Appropriate management, a sound knowledge of angiology and cooperation between healthcare professionals are essential to ensure effective treatment and a better quality of life for those affected.

Endovascular and techniques minimally invasive

Looking back over the history of vascular surgery, it is fascinating to see how technology and techniques have evolved. From major incisions and long recovery periods, we have moved on to procedures where the patient can often leave hospital on the same day as the operation. Endovascular and minimally invasive techniques are perfect examples of this, offering less traumatic solutions with often superior results.

1. What is endovascular surgery?
   - Definition and basic principles
   - Developments in surgical techniques
   - Advantages over traditional open surgery
2. Minimally invasive techniques: a brief introduction
   - Mini-invasive" concept
   - Main techniques: angioplasty, stenting, ablation
   - Developments in medical devices
3. Materials and preparation :
   - Catheters, guidewires and stents
   - Imaging: the importance of angiography and fluoroscopy
   - Preparing the patient and the surgical site
4. Common interventions and their indications :
   - **Angioplasty**: dilation of a narrowed or blocked blood vessel
   - **Stenting** : A device used to keep a vessel open.
   - **Embolisation**: targeted blockage of a blood vessel
   - Ablation by radiofrequency or laser : Treatment of varicose veins
5. Advantages and benefits :
   - Less post-operative pain
   - Faster recovery and shorter hospital stays
   - Reduced risk of infection and complications
   - Superior aesthetic results with small incisions
6. Limitations and challenges :
   - Not suitable for all patients or conditions
   - Need for specific training and specialised equipment
   - Management of potential complications
7. The future of minimally invasive techniques :
   - Innovations in medical equipment and devices

- Emerging techniques: robotics and computer-aided navigation
- Training and education: preparing the next generation of vascular surgeons

The evolution of endovascular surgery and minimally invasive techniques is a perfect example of how medical science continues to advance to offer patients better, less invasive and more effective care. While recognising the immense benefits, it is crucial to continue to train, adapt and innovate to meet the future challenges of vascular surgery.

The role of the nurse in cardiovascular surgery

Cardiovascular surgery is complex and often urgent, requiring a multidisciplinary approach in which every member of the medical team plays a crucial role. Nurses are the linchpin of this team, with responsibilities that go well beyond basic nursing care. Understanding the scope of these responsibilities helps to emphasise the importance of their role in the success of cardiovascular interventions.

1. Preoperative preparation :
    - **Initial assessment of the patient:** medical history, preliminary examinations, current medications.
    - **Patient education:** Explanation of the procedure, risks, recovery process.
    - **Coordination with the team:** Ensuring smooth communication between surgeons, anaesthetists and other healthcare professionals.
2. Assistance during the operation :
    - **Patient monitoring:** constant monitoring of vital signs, heart rate and other essential parameters.

- **Equipment management:** Preparation and sterilisation of instruments, anticipation of the surgeon's needs.
- **Team support:** Ongoing communication with the team to ensure smooth operations.

3. Post-operative management :
   - **Continuous monitoring:** monitoring vital signs, early detection of possible complications.
   - **Pain management:** administering analgesic drugs, assessing their effectiveness and adjusting doses.
   - **Education and support:** Helping patients to understand their condition, the after-effects of surgery, rehabilitation and the follow-up plan.

4. Rehabilitation and long-term follow-up :
   - **Orientation:** Working with physiotherapists and other professionals to rehabilitate the patient's heart.
   - **Regular monitoring:** ensuring medical follow-up, monitoring medication side-effects and adjusting treatments.

5. Emotional and psychological role :
   - **Emotional support:** listening to patients and their families, offering psychological support in times of stress and uncertainty.
   - **Advocacy:** Defending patients' rights, ensuring that their concerns are heard and taken into account.

6. Further training and specialisation :
   - **Keeping your skills up to date:** attending training courses and conferences, and keeping abreast of the latest advances in cardiovascular surgery.
   - **Specialisation:** Some nurses may choose to specialise in specific areas such as cardiac intensive care or paediatric cardiac surgery.

The cardiovascular surgery nurse does more than just provide care; he or she is a fundamental part of the medical team. Their role, which encompasses technical skills, emotion, education and coordination, is essential to guaranteeing the patient's well-being and the success of the operation. In an ever-changing medical world, the nurse remains the guarantor of holistic care, combining competence, compassion and dedication.

Chapter 25:
PATIENT SAFETY AND MANAGEMENT MEDICAL ERRORS

Preventing errors in vascular surgery

In surgery, where the margins for error are often tiny, error prevention is of paramount importance. In vascular surgery, given the complexity of the procedures and the fragility of the vascular systems involved, this prevention is particularly important. The consequences of an error can be serious, ranging from post-operative complications to lasting or even fatal after-effects.

1. Training and education :
The first step in preventing errors is to ensure solid, ongoing training for surgeons and all medical staff. This includes learning surgical techniques, becoming familiar with equipment and constantly updating knowledge.

2. Pre-operative planning :
Careful planning is crucial to avoid errors. This includes a review of the patient's medical history, radiological examinations and team discussion of the best surgical strategies.

3. Checklists:
Inspired by the aeronautics industry, checklists in surgery have proved their effectiveness in reducing errors. Before starting an operation, the team goes through a checklist, making sure that all the pre-operative steps have been followed.

4. Open communication :
Fluid and transparent communication within the medical team is fundamental. Each member must feel free to report a problem, ask a question or seek clarification.

5. Advanced technologies :
The use of modern technologies, such as robot-assisted surgery or enhanced visualisation systems, can help minimise errors.

6. Morbidity and mortality reviews:
These are regular meetings at which medical teams discuss complex cases, complications or errors, in a spirit of training and continuous improvement.

7. Patient feedback:
Feedback from patients and their families can provide valuable information for identifying areas for improvement.

8. Compliance with protocols :
Protocols and guidelines are there for a reason. They are based on scientific evidence and must be strictly followed to ensure patient safety.

9. Emergency training :
Errors are more likely to occur in stressful situations. Training in emergency situations, through simulations or specific courses, can help the team to react better to these situations.

Preventing errors in vascular surgery is an ongoing process, requiring the active participation of every member of the medical team. It is by combining training, communication, technology and critical thinking that patient safety will be ensured and standards of care will be consistently high.

Managing and communicating after an error

Medical error is a sensitive and painful subject, both for carers and patients. The stakes are even higher in vascular surgery, where the margins for error are slim and the consequences potentially far-reaching. The post-medical error phase is therefore a critical time when it is essential to demonstrate tact, transparency and humanity.

1. Immediate recognition of the error :
The first and often most difficult step is to acknowledge that the error has occurred. This requires introspection, an acceptance of human fallibility, and a willingness not to ignore or conceal the error.

2. Open communication with patients and their families:
Patients have the right to know what happened. The discussion should be honest, clear and compassionate. Avoid medical jargon and be prepared to answer questions and concerns.

3. Ensure the patient's immediate safety :
Above all, it is crucial to ensure that the patient is safe and to take all necessary steps to remedy the error or minimise its effects.

4. Analysis of the error :
To prevent the error from happening again, it is essential to understand how and why it occurred. This may require an in-depth analysis, involving the entire medical team and sometimes an external expert.

5. Liability and redress :
Taking responsibility for the mistake is crucial. This can include a sincere apology, compensation if necessary, and above all, a guarantee that steps are being taken to prevent it happening again.

6. Psychological support for the medical team :
A medical error can be traumatic for healthcare staff. It is essential to offer support, whether in the form of debriefing, counselling or psychological follow-up.

7. Training and prevention :
Following an error, it is crucial to invest in training and updating the skills of the team. This can also be an opportunity to review and adjust existing protocols.

8. Institutional transparency :
Healthcare institutions have a role to play in encouraging a

culture of transparency. This can take the form of incident reports, morbidity and mortality reviews or training sessions.

9. Rebuilding trust :
After a mistake, it is natural for the trust between the patient and the medical team to be shaken. Rebuilding it will take time, listening and constant communication.

Managing and communicating after an error is a delicate challenge that tests the integrity, humanity and professionalism of carers. By focusing on transparency, empathy and prevention, it is possible to transform these painful moments into opportunities for learning and growth.

Feedback for continuous improvement

In the dynamic and complex world of vascular surgery, every patient, every case, is a mine of valuable information. Every situation, whether successful or not, is a learning opportunity. Feedback is emerging as a powerful strategy for consolidating this learning, enabling medical teams to constantly improve.

1. Understanding feedback :
Feedback is the systematic analysis of an event, situation or process. It aims to identify what worked well, what could have been done differently and what lessons can be learned.

2. Sources of feedback :
They can arise from a variety of situations: a particularly complex operation, an unexpected incident, the introduction of a new technology or technique, or even a simple day-to-day exchange with a patient.

3. Setting up a feedback system :

- **Gathering information:** Through interviews, post-operative debriefings, team meetings, or even anonymous surveys.
- **Analysis and interpretation:** look for trends, identify root causes and highlight areas for improvement.
- **Implementing actions:** This can range from additional training to the modification of certain protocols, via the acquisition of new equipment.

4. Foster an open culture :

For REX to be effective, we need to encourage a culture where staff feel safe to share their opinions, concerns and mistakes without fear of repercussions.

5. Feedback and continuing training:

The lessons learned from feedback can enrich continuing training programmes, making them more relevant and adapted to the reality on the ground.

6. Communicating feedback :

It is essential to share the results of feedback with the whole team, and sometimes even beyond, with other establishments or in specialist publications.

7. Feedback and technology :

As technology evolves, specialist software can help to collect, analyse and share feedback effectively.

8. The limits of REX :

Although powerful, REX has its limits. They require time, resources and constant commitment. What's more, without proper implementation of corrective actions, feedback can lose its relevance.

Feedback is more than just a post-facto analysis. It embodies the spirit of modern medicine, which is proactive and focused on continuous improvement. By capitalising on each experience, vascular surgery can not only improve the quality of care, but also strengthen the trust between carers and patients.

Chapter 26:
RESOURCE MANAGEMENT AND OPERATIONAL EFFICIENCY

Optimising patient flows and the use of resources

In the hospital environment, and more particularly in vascular surgery, optimising patient flows and the use of resources has become imperative. Faced with increasing demands, tight budgets and evolving technologies, optimal management not only makes for greater efficiency, but also improves the quality of care. Let's decipher together how to navigate this complex issue.

1. Analysis of current patient flows :
First and foremost, it is vital to understand how things currently work. This involves a detailed analysis of the patient pathway, from admission to discharge, identifying potential bottlenecks, waiting times and redundancies.

2. The importance of triage :
Effective triage can significantly improve patient flow. In vascular surgery, this means quickly identifying the severity and complexity of cases, so that patients can be directed to the right contacts or procedures.

3. Interdisciplinary coordination :
Close collaboration between surgeons, nurses, anaesthetists, radiologists and other specialists is crucial. Fluid communication helps to avoid delays, reduce length of stay and improve overall management.

4. Optimal management of equipment and operating theatres :
The efficient use of operating theatres, imaging equipment and other resources can greatly influence patient flow. This

requires rigorous planning, preventive maintenance and flexibility in the event of emergencies.

5. Training and education :
Investing in ongoing staff training is essential. A well-trained team, up to date with the latest techniques and protocols, is better able to manage patients effectively while optimising the resources available.

6. The contribution of technology :
Modern hospital information systems can help to monitor patient flow in real time, anticipate resource requirements and adjust schedules accordingly.

7. Feedback and continuous improvement:
As mentioned above, it is essential to learn from each situation in order to improve. Feedback from patients, families and professionals provides opportunities to adjust and refine processes.

8. Patient awareness and education:
A well-informed patient, who understands the stages of his or her journey, is more inclined to cooperate, thus reducing delays and unforeseen events.

Optimising patient flow and the use of resources is a major challenge, but one that is essential if we are to meet the challenges facing vascular surgery today. By adopting a holistic, patient-centred approach and using modern tools and technologies, it is possible to offer high-quality care while effectively managing the resources available.

Time management techniques and workload

Managing time and workload is an ever-present challenge, especially in demanding environments such as healthcare. Knowing how to navigate these challenges effectively not only improves productivity, but also preserves mental health and well-being. Let's take a look at some key techniques for achieving this.

1. Prioritising tasks :
This is often the first step. Identify which tasks are urgent, which can wait and which can be delegated. Using the Eisenhower matrix, which ranks tasks according to their urgency and importance, can be useful.

2. Planning:
Start each day or week with a clearly defined list of tasks. Use tools such as diaries, digital calendars or task management applications to help you.

3. Time blocks :
Divide your day into dedicated blocks of time. For example, set aside an hour to answer emails, then another for consultations, and so on. This limits interruptions and allows you to concentrate fully on one task at a time.

4. The two-minute rule:
If a task can be done in less than two minutes, do it immediately. This avoids accumulating small tasks that can quickly become overwhelming.

5. Learning to say no :
It's important to recognise your limits. If you already have a heavy workload, it's legitimate to refuse additional tasks or to ask for support.

6. Delegation :
Don't fall into the trap of wanting to do everything yourself. Identify tasks that can be delegated and entrust them to colleagues or competent subordinates.

7. Take breaks:
There's evidence that short but regular breaks can increase productivity and reduce stress. Whether it's a brisk walk, a few minutes' meditation or simply getting away from your desk, these breaks are crucial.

8. Avoid multitasking:
Contrary to popular belief, multitasking can reduce

efficiency and increase errors. Concentrate on one task at a time, finish it, then move on to the next.

9. Minimise distractions:
Put your phone on silent mode, close unnecessary tabs on your computer and create a working environment conducive to concentration.

10. Ongoing training :
Invest time in training to learn new management techniques or tools that can help you be more efficient.

Time and workload management is an art that requires practice, adaptability and perseverance. By adopting a structured approach and remaining aware of your limits, you can achieve a healthy balance between professional efficiency and personal well-being.

Technology as an efficiency tool

Throughout the ages, technology has always been a catalyst for progress. In the medical field, it has become an indispensable tool for increasing efficiency, improving patient care and pushing back the boundaries of what medicine can achieve.

1. Rapid, accurate diagnosis:
Advances in medical imaging, particularly with CT, MRI and ultrasound, have transformed diagnosis. These tools offer a clear view of the inside of the body, enabling the detection of diseases that were previously difficult to identify.

2. Telemedicine:
The possibility of consulting at a distance, particularly in remote areas or in pandemic situations, has made healthcare more accessible. Telemedicine also reduces the cost and travel time for patients.

3. Simulations and virtual reality:
These tools enable healthcare professionals to practise

performing procedures without risk to the patient, thereby increasing competence and reducing errors.

4. Connected objects:
From smartwatches to monitoring devices, these gadgets collect data in real time, offering a constant snapshot of an individual's health. This information can be used to adapt treatments and for prevention.

5. Robotic surgery:
Systems such as the Da Vinci allow surgeons to perform operations with greater precision, minimising incisions, reducing recovery time and increasing success rates.

6. Artificial intelligence:
AI is used to rapidly analyse large volumes of data, aid diagnosis, predict epidemics, and even advise on treatment plans.

7. Information sharing platforms :
Electronic medical record systems facilitate collaboration between healthcare professionals and ensure that all relevant information is easily accessible.

8. 3D printing:
From creating personalised prostheses to printing organic tissue, 3D printing offers innovative solutions to medical challenges.

Technology, as a tool for efficiency, has profoundly transformed medicine. It has opened doors that were previously unthinkable, improving quality of life and life expectancy. But with these benefits also come challenges, particularly in terms of ethics, safety and training. It is essential that healthcare professionals keep abreast of these advances, while bearing in mind the paramount importance of the human aspect of care.

Chapter 27:
THE FUTURE OF VASCULAR SURGERY : SCENARIOS AND PROJECTIONS

Technological advances on the horizon

As technology advances, medicine continues to evolve at an unprecedented rate. Innovations once relegated to the realms of science fiction are now within reach. Here's a look at the technological advances that could shape the medical landscape of tomorrow.

1. Nanotechnology:
The ability to manipulate materials on a molecular scale opens new doors for the precise targeting of drugs, the treatment of tumours and even the repair of damaged cells.
2. 3D bioprinting:
Beyond printing prostheses, the prospect of printing functional human organs could revolutionise transplantation and put an end to the organ shortage.
3. Gene therapies and CRISPR:
The ability to modify the human genome could not only treat but also prevent a wide range of genetic diseases, while raising major ethical debates.
4. Augmented reality and surgery:
Augmented reality glasses or lenses could provide surgeons with real-time information during operations, improving accuracy and reducing risk.
5. Advanced artificial intelligence:
Beyond diagnostics, AI could play a role in personalising treatment plans, predicting epidemics and even delivering care directly in certain scenarios.
6. Brain-Computer Interface (BCI) systems:
The ability to connect the brain directly to machines could offer revolutionary solutions for the paralysed, people

suffering from neurological disorders or even to improve cognitive abilities.

7. Advanced robotics:
AI-assisted robots could one day perform surgery without human intervention, look after post-operative patients or assist the elderly in their own homes.

8. Next-generation wearables :
Even more advanced wearable devices, capable of continuously monitoring a multitude of health parameters, could predict medical problems before they even occur.

9. Personalised treatments:
By combining genomics and metabolomics, medicine could be perfectly tailored to the individual, maximising effectiveness and minimising side effects.

10. Alternative energies in medicine:
The exploration of methods such as optogenetics, where nerve cells are controlled by light, is opening up exciting avenues for the treatment of neurological diseases.

These advances, while promising, will also bring their share of challenges, particularly in terms of regulation, ethics and safety. But one thing is certain: the future of medicine looks bright, with almost limitless possibilities for improving quality of life and extending life expectancy.

Demographic challenges and epidemiological data

In an ever-changing world, demographic and epidemiological challenges have a profound influence on healthcare systems and the delivery of care. These challenges are shaping not only how governments, institutions and healthcare professionals interact, but also how they plan for the future.

1. The ageing of the population :
Many parts of the world, particularly developed countries, are facing an increase in the number of elderly people. This is leading to increased demand for chronic healthcare, rising medical costs, and the need to adapt infrastructures and services to the needs of the elderly.

2. Epidemiological transition:
We are seeing a transition from infectious diseases to non-communicable diseases such as cardiovascular disease, diabetes and cancer. This requires a change in the training of health professionals, medical research and prevention policies.

3. Increasing urbanisation :
Migration to urban areas leads to increased population density, which can facilitate the spread of infectious diseases. In addition, urban living is associated with an increase in lifestyle-related diseases such as obesity.

4. Antibiotic resistance :
The overuse and misuse of antibiotics has led to an increase in resistance, making some previously treatable diseases much harder to combat.

5. Inequalities in health :
Despite medical advances, major health disparities persist between rich and poor countries, and even within countries themselves. These inequalities can be exacerbated by socio-economic, cultural and political factors.

6. Migratory movements:
Migration flows, whether voluntary or forced, can introduce new diseases to regions and challenge local health systems.

7. Environmental change and health:
Climate change, deforestation and urbanisation can increase the risk of epidemics of diseases such as malaria, dengue fever and Zika. They can also have indirect effects, such as malnutrition due to disruption of food chains.

8. New epidemics and pandemics:
The threat of new emerging diseases, such as COVID-19,

highlights the need for global epidemiological surveillance and pandemic preparedness.

In the face of these challenges, global collaboration, long-term planning and investment in research and development are essential. Policy-makers, researchers and health professionals must work together to anticipate, understand and respond to these challenges, to ensure a healthy future for all.

Looking ahead : preparing the nurse of tomorrow

As the medical landscape evolves, the role of the nurse is changing and adapting, reflecting advances in technology, new methods of care and changing patient expectations. To effectively prepare the nurse of tomorrow, it is essential to take these future trends and challenges into account.

1. The age of digitalisation:
The growing adoption of telemedicine, electronic medical records and connected objects will require skills in health technology. Tomorrow's nurse will need to be comfortable with these tools, ensuring that they are used effectively and that patient data is secure.

2. Holistic approach to care:
Rather than focusing solely on treating symptoms, the modern nurse must adopt a more holistic approach, taking into account all of the patient's needs - physical, emotional, social and mental.

3. Continuing education:
With medical protocols, drugs and technologies constantly evolving, continuous learning will be essential. The ability to learn and adapt quickly will become a key skill.

4. Increased specialisation:
Like doctors, nurses could become more specialised,

offering expert care in areas such as vascular surgery, oncology or paediatrics.

5. A more autonomous role:
In many regions, particularly in the face of a shortage of doctors, nurses can take on greater responsibilities, such as prescribing medicines or carrying out certain procedures.

6. Interdisciplinary collaboration:
Tomorrow's nurse will work even more closely with a diverse team of healthcare professionals, social workers and even engineers or designers, to deliver innovative and integrated care.

7. Ethics and humanism :
With the advent of technologies such as genomics or artificial intelligence in medicine, nurses will have to navigate complex ethical waters, always placing patients' needs and rights at the centre of their concerns.

8. Crisis preparedness :
Recent pandemics have highlighted the crucial role of nurses on the front line. Solid training in crisis management, trauma psychology and emergency care will be essential.

Tomorrow's nurse will be technologically savvy, specialised and autonomous, but will remain deeply rooted in the humanistic and ethical values of the profession. To ensure that nurses are ready to meet these challenges, educational institutions, regulatory bodies and hospitals must anticipate these developments and offer appropriate training and support.

Chapter 28:
PROFESSIONAL DEVELOPMENT

Continuing education and specialisation

In the ever-changing world of medicine, continuing education and specialisation are not only desirable, they are becoming an imperative necessity. With the emergence of new technologies, the constant expansion of knowledge and the changing needs of patients, healthcare professionals, including nurses, are under constant pressure to remain at the cutting edge of their field.

Continuing education enables nurses to keep abreast of the latest advances in care, acquire new skills and meet the high standards of the profession. It plays a key role not only in improving clinical skills, but also in boosting patient confidence and professional satisfaction. It is through continuous updating of their knowledge that nurses can deliver high-quality, evidence-based care and best practice.

Alongside continuing education, specialisation has become a path increasingly taken by many nurses. Whether it's vascular surgery, oncology, intensive care or mental health, specialising allows nurses to deepen their knowledge in a specific field. This in-depth expertise translates into better patient care and often into greater professional recognition.

Specialisation not only offers advantages in terms of skills. It also offers the opportunity to work closely with other specialists, to have access to cutting-edge technologies and to participate in innovative research in specific fields. What's more, it can open the door to leadership, training or consultancy roles.

But continuing training and specialisation are not without their challenges. Further training requires time, financial resources and personal commitment. It's an investment in itself. Yet the benefits in terms of improved patient care, personal satisfaction and career progression are inestimable.

Continuing education and specialisation are essential steps for any healthcare professional wishing to offer the best to their patients and to develop their career. In a world where change is the only constant, adapting and evolving is the way to stay relevant and effective.

Interdisciplinary collaboration

The medical world is a complex web of knowledge, skills and expertise. Each branch of medicine has its own particularities, specialists and methods. However, in the vast world of medicine, it has become imperative for these different branches to be able to collaborate, exchange ideas and work together for the benefit of the patient. This is where interdisciplinary collaboration really comes into its own.

Interdisciplinary collaboration is an integrated approach in which various healthcare professionals from different disciplines come together around a patient or clinical case to provide holistic care. In the context of vascular surgery, for example, a patient might require the intervention of a vascular surgeon, a cardiologist, a radiologist and, of course, a specialist nurse, to name but a few.

These collaborations are all the more essential given that vascular pathologies are often multifactorial. A diabetic patient, for example, could have renal, cardiac and vascular complications. In such cases, teamwork between different specialists makes it possible to design and implement a personalised care plan that is effective and tailored to the complexity of the case.

But beyond clinical care, these collaborations also have a significant impact on training and research. Exchanges between professionals from different disciplines encourage the sharing of knowledge, the emergence of new ideas and the questioning of existing practices. This synergy is the breeding ground for medical innovations and discoveries that will shape the medicine of tomorrow.

However, interdisciplinary collaboration is not without its challenges. It requires open communication, mutual trust, and a willingness to share and learn. Each professional must recognise the value and expertise of the other members of the team and be prepared to put egos aside for the good of the patient.

For nurses, this collaboration is also an invaluable opportunity for learning and professional development. It enables them to gain a better understanding of the different facets of a clinical case, hone their skills and broaden their field of knowledge.

Interdisciplinary collaboration is an essential pillar of modern medicine. They symbolise a medicine that recognises the complexity of the human body and the need for an integrated approach to meet today's medical challenges. For patients, it's a guarantee of comprehensive, high-quality care, where every aspect of their health is taken into account. For professionals, it's an invitation to grow, to learn and, together, to build the medicine of tomorrow.

Research and academic contributions

Medicine, in its constant quest for improvement, is intrinsically linked to academic research. Academic research is the foundation on which new discoveries, technological innovations and therapeutic advances are built. In the field of vascular surgery, as in so many other medical disciplines, academic research and contributions play a cardinal role.

Vascular surgery research encompasses a variety of fields, from the molecular understanding of vascular diseases to the development of new surgical techniques. Every study, every article published, every clinical trial contributes to enriching our understanding of the discipline and refining treatment methods.

Academic contributions in this sector are many and varied. They may involve the study of new vascular prostheses, the development of more precise imaging techniques, the design of less invasive surgical protocols, or the discovery of therapeutic molecules to prevent thrombus formation.

Nurses, although on the front line of clinical care, also have a role to play in this research. Their practical experience, direct contact with patients and daily observation of post-operative results make them a valuable source of information. Increasingly, nurses are becoming involved in research projects, sharing their observations, taking part in clinical studies, or even initiating their own research.

Academic contributions are not limited to the laboratory or operating theatre. Medical conferences, seminars, workshops and publications enable the medical community to stay at the cutting edge of knowledge, share best practice and debate the latest innovations. These platforms are essential to ensure evidence-based medicine, where every intervention and every decision is supported by solid scientific data.

Research and academic contributions are the driving force behind medical progress. In a world where diseases are evolving, where patients are increasingly well-informed and demanding, and where technology is advancing at a breathtaking pace, it is imperative that vascular surgery, like all medical disciplines, continues to renew itself, to question itself and to progress. It is this quest for knowledge, this desire to constantly improve care, that guarantees today's and tomorrow's patients high-quality, effective and humane medicine.

Conclusion:
THE FUTURE OF VASCULAR SURGERY AND THE ROLE OF THE NURSE

Technological advances and innovations

At the dawn of the 21st century, vascular surgery has seen unprecedented technological advances, pushing back the boundaries of what is possible and revolutionising patient care. These innovations, combined with a better understanding of vascular pathologies, have paved the way for more precise, less invasive procedures with higher success rates.

One of the major innovations in this field is the advent of endovascular surgery. Unlike traditional open surgery, this technique uses small catheters inserted into the blood vessels, allowing the surgeon to operate without large incisions. As a result, patients benefit from shorter recovery times, reduced post-operative risks and minimal scarring.

Medical imaging, with technologies such as MRI angiography and computed tomography angiography (CT angiography), now offers high-resolution visualisations of blood vessels. These techniques not only allow vascular anomalies to be detected and diagnosed with precision, but also enable endovascular interventions to be guided in real time.

Advances in biomedical materials have also played a crucial role. Stents have been optimised to be more flexible, durable and biocompatible. New antithrombotic materials reduce the risk of clot formation, while drug-eluting stents slowly release drugs to prevent restenosis.

Surgical robotics, although still in its infancy in vascular surgery, promises even more precise and standardised interventions. Guided by artificial intelligence and advanced vision systems, surgical robots can access hard-to-reach areas and perform movements with unrivalled precision.

Telemedicine, reinforced by the increasing digitalisation of healthcare, offers another remarkable advance. It enables remote monitoring of patients, especially in remote areas, guaranteeing continuity of post-operative care and rapid intervention in the event of any anomaly.

Finally, the growing adoption of digital twin systems, which create a digital replica of patients' vascular systems, could offer surgeons a simulation platform for planning and performing complex procedures.

These innovations, the result of a combination of clinical research, biomedical engineering and cutting-edge technology, illustrate the rapid evolution of vascular surgery. With these advances, the future of the specialty looks bright, offering the hope of even more effective and safer treatments for patients around the world.

Evolution of the nursing role in a changing medical world

The medical world is constantly evolving, driven by technological advances, scientific discoveries and socio-economic and demographic challenges. At the heart of this dynamic, the role of the nurse, traditionally seen as a support worker, is also undergoing profound change, becoming more diversified and taking on greater responsibilities.

Historically, nurses were often seen as the doctor's right-hand man, with a role focused on patient care, listening and well-being. However, with the increasing complexity of care, the need for multidisciplinary patient management and legislative changes, nurses are now a central link in the medical system.

The expansion of advanced nursing practice is a striking illustration of this. In many countries, nurse practitioners can now make diagnoses, prescribe medicines and manage medical cases independently. This development not only reflects the recognition of nursing skills, but also responds to the need to optimise patient care, particularly in regions with a shortage of doctors.

The digitalisation of care is another vector for change. The modern nurse has to navigate in an environment where telemedicine, electronic medical records and connected objects are ubiquitous. This requires continuous training and adaptability in the face of new technologies, but in return offers the ability to monitor patients in a more precise and personalised way.
The management of chronicity, with the increase in chronic illnesses, has also rethought the nursing role. Rather than focusing solely on acute care, nurses now play a major role in long-term monitoring, therapeutic education and prevention.

Demographic challenges, particularly the ageing of the population, accentuate the need for a holistic approach to care where the nurse goes beyond medical care to take account of the psychosocial dimension, mental well-being and maintaining autonomy.

What's more, given the growing complexity of care pathways, nurses are becoming essential coordinators, facilitating communication between specialists, paramedics and patients, guaranteeing continuity of care and optimised management.

These developments are accompanied by an enhancement of nursing training, greater recognition of their expertise and greater autonomy in their practice.

Today's nurse is at the crossroads of medical, technological and social issues. In a medical world undergoing constant change, nurses are more than ever a central figure, versatile and essential to the well-being of patients.

Advice for aspiring nurses in vascular surgery

Vascular surgery is an exciting but demanding area of medicine. For those who aspire to become nurses in this sector, here are some tips on how to get started and excel in this speciality:

- **Solid training**: Make sure you get quality training, ideally from a recognised institution. In addition to general nursing training, consider taking specialised courses in vascular surgery.
- **Practical experience**: Try to get internships or junior positions in vascular surgery departments. Field experience is invaluable in understanding the nuances of this specialty.
- **Keep up to date**: Medicine is changing fast. Attend seminars, workshops and conferences. Subscribe to specialist journals to keep abreast of the latest developments.
- **Professional network**: Connect with experienced professionals in the field. They can offer you advice, recommendations and perhaps even professional opportunities.

- **Interpersonal skills**: In vascular surgery, you will work with patients, surgeons, anaesthetists and other members of the medical team. Good communication skills are essential to ensure quality care.
- **Stress management**: Working in vascular surgery can be stressful, with frequent emergencies. Learn how to manage stress, whether through relaxation techniques, meditation or other methods.
- **Continuity of care**: Vascular surgery doesn't stop in the operating theatre. Make sure you understand the importance of post-operative follow-up and pay attention to your patients' needs after the operation.
- **Professional ethics**: Always respect the nursing code of ethics. Integrity, confidentiality and commitment to patients are paramount.
- **Specialisation**: Consider deepening your skills with an additional specialisation or certification, such as vascular ultrasound or vascular surgical intensive care.
- **Passion and dedication**: As with any medical profession, having a real passion for what you do can make all the difference. Dedication to your profession and to your patients will help you overcome challenges and find satisfaction in your work.

Entering the field of vascular surgery as a nurse is a major commitment, but with determination, the right training and a genuine desire to help others, it can be an extremely rewarding career.

Made in the USA
Monee, IL
14 January 2025

76874670R00095